10

AF771389

PHARMACOLOGY - RESEARCH, SAFETY TESTING AND REGULATION

CLOPIDOGREL

PHARMACOLOGY, CLINICAL USES AND ADVERSE EFFECTS

PHARMACOLOGY - RESEARCH, SAFETY TESTING AND REGULATION

Additional books in this series can be found on Nova's website under the Series tab.

Additional e-books in this series can be found on Nova's website under the e-book tab.

PHARMACOLOGY - RESEARCH, SAFETY TESTING AND REGULATION

CLOPIDOGREL

PHARMACOLOGY, CLINICAL USES AND ADVERSE EFFECTS

JAMES P. ALESCI
AND
ALEXANDER VICTORINO
EDITORS

NOVA BIOMEDICAL

New York

Copyright © 2014 by Nova Science Publishers, Inc.

All rights reserved. No part of this book may be reproduced, stored in a retrieval system or transmitted in any form or by any means: electronic, electrostatic, magnetic, tape, mechanical photocopying, recording or otherwise without the written permission of the Publisher.

For permission to use material from this book please contact us:
Telephone 631-231-7269; Fax 631-231-8175
Web Site: http://www.novapublishers.com

NOTICE TO THE READER

The Publisher has taken reasonable care in the preparation of this book, but makes no expressed or implied warranty of any kind and assumes no responsibility for any errors or omissions. No liability is assumed for incidental or consequential damages in connection with or arising out of information contained in this book. The Publisher shall not be liable for any special, consequential, or exemplary damages resulting, in whole or in part, from the readers' use of, or reliance upon, this material. Any parts of this book based on government reports are so indicated and copyright is claimed for those parts to the extent applicable to compilations of such works.

Independent verification should be sought for any data, advice or recommendations contained in this book. In addition, no responsibility is assumed by the publisher for any injury and/or damage to persons or property arising from any methods, products, instructions, ideas or otherwise contained in this publication.

This publication is designed to provide accurate and authoritative information with regard to the subject matter covered herein. It is sold with the clear understanding that the Publisher is not engaged in rendering legal or any other professional services. If legal or any other expert assistance is required, the services of a competent person should be sought. FROM A DECLARATION OF PARTICIPANTS JOINTLY ADOPTED BY A COMMITTEE OF THE AMERICAN BAR ASSOCIATION AND A COMMITTEE OF PUBLISHERS.

Additional color graphics may be available in the e-book version of this book.

Library of Congress Cataloging-in-Publication Data

ISBN: 978-1-62948-336-8

Library of Congress Control Number: 2013950570

Published by Nova Science Publishers, Inc. † New York

Contents

Preface

Clopidogrel is an oral thienopyridine derivative, used as an anti-platelet aggregation agent to inhibit blood clot formation in coronary artery disease, peripheral vascular disease and cerebrovascular disease. In this book, the authors discuss the pharmacology, clinical uses and adverse effects of clopidogrel. Topics include clopidogrel use in neurointerventional surgery; management of clopidogrel hypersensitivity; clopidogrel and gastrointestinal harm; perioperative management of clopidogrel in urological surgery; and platelet function testing to guide therapy in poor responders to clopidogrel.

Chapter 1 - Warfarin was the mainstay of oral anticoagulant therapy until the recent discovery of more precise targets for therapy. Although warfarin therapy is plagued by a narrow therapeutic index, variable individual metabolic responses, and numerous food and drug interactions, newer agents purport to rise above these setbacks. Furthermore, while the safety of these new drugs compared to traditional therapy has been called into question, their ease of use makes it unlikely that they will disappear.

This review will explore the mechanisms of action and pharmacokinetics of traditional and novel anticoagulants and antiplatelet agents. In addition, recommended withholding periods for these drugs for patients undergoing elective endoscopic procedures as well as options for achieving rapid hemostasis in patients undergoing emergent endoscopy.

Chapter 2 - Neurointerventional surgery has become an essential tool for the treatment of complex spinal and cerebrovascular diseases including cerebral aneurysms, dural arteriovenous fistulas (dAVF), arteriovenous malformations (AVM), carotid-cavernous fistulas, intra/extracranial atherosclerosis, intracranial thromboembolism, and neurological tumors. Techniques utilizing stents, coils, neuroembolic agents, flow-diverting devices, and combinations thereof are often used to treat these diverse pathologies. While significant advances have been made in the field of neurointerventional surgery in recent years, the risk of peri-procedural thromboembolic complications (e.g., transient ischemic attack [TIA] and ischemic stroke) has been estimated at 8% due to the thrombogenic nature of the foreign guidewires and endovascular implants. Interventional cardiology—a field that utilizes similar endovascular techniques for stenting of diseased coronary vessels in myocardial ischemia/infarction—has demonstrated that post-procedural dual anti-platelet therapy (DAPT) with aspirin and clopidogrel minimizes the risk of thromboembolic complications and is more beneficial than aspirin therapy alone. Due to these findings, DAPT with aspirin (325 mg PO daily) and clopidogrel (75 mg PO daily), with or without a loading dose, has been recommended for neurointerventional procedures as well. However, limited research on the use of aspirin and clopidogrel for neurointerventional surgery currently exists in the literature to support these recommendations, and there are no formal guidelines for the use of anti-platelet agents in this setting. Additionally, recent data suggest that a large number of patients exhibit clopidogrel resistance, which may increase the rate of thromboembolic complications during endovascular procedures. As a result, novel anti-platelet agents are being increasingly utilized in this challenging patient population. The goal of this chapter is to highlight the use of clopidogrel in neurointerventional surgery, including indications for treatment, complications of treatment, challenges to the current treatment paradigm, methods for detection, and possible anti-platelet alternatives.

Chapter 3 - In 1998 the European Commission granted the first marketing authorization for the potent anti-platelet aggregation agent clopidogrel to Sanofi Pharma Bristol-Myers Squibb SNC; the pharmacokinetic section of the Scientific Discussion which was part of the European Public Assessment Report stated that plasma levels of the parent compound beyond 2 hours from administration are very low, below the quantification limit of the existing method, and the only pharmacokinetic information available were on the inactive clopidogrel carboxylic metabolite. Clopidogrel appeared from the beginning to be a prodrug; however, detailed information on the chemical structure and pharmacology of the active moiety, the thiol metabolite responsible of the therapeutic action, were only published in 2000, leaving in any case open the discussion on the pharmacokinetic aspects of this molecule. Four years later, in 2004, the first clopidogrel pharmacokinetic data in man was presented and, in the same year, the first paper on the determination of clopidogrel active metabolite in plasma was published. It is noteworthy that for many years the analytical methods aiming to quantify clopidogrel in human plasma have encountered big problems. Until in 2010, a more clear understanding of the problem was reached, discovering that a new metabolite of clopidogrel is responsible for back-conversion to clopidogrel during sample handling. In the same years the oxidative steps involved in the synthesis of the active metabolite were studied and cytochrome P450 isoenzymes 2B6, 3A4, 1A1, 1A2 and 2C19 were identified as the most important. As a result of these findings, and of several PK/PD and genotype studies, in 2010, the FDA approved a new label for clopidogrel with a "boxed warning" about the diminished effectiveness of the drug in patients with impaired ability to convert the prodrug into its active form. Meanwhile a lot of progress was done also in the identification and quantitation of other clopidogrel metabolites like oxo-clopidogrel and clopidogrel acyl-glucuronide. Despite 15 years have passed from the introduction of clopidogrel in the market, the pharmacokinetic of this molecule still intrigues and attracts the attention of the scientific community.

Chapter 4 - Clopidogrel is widely used to treat acute coronary syndromes (ACS) and peripheral vascular diseases, particularly among patients undergoing percutaneous coronary intervention (PCI). It is the therapeutic agent of choice to prevent thrombotic events associated with cardiovascular stenting. However nearly 20-40% patients respond poorly to the standard regimen of clopidogrel therapy and these patients are at increased risk for ischemic complications and cardiovascular deaths. Although there are intensive efforts to search for genetic markers for this interindividual variability in clopidogrel therapy, results have been mixed and inconclusive. Based on the mechanistic studies of clopidogrel metabolism, it is most likely that the interindividual variability in clopidogrel therapy is multifactorial. A crucial factor contributing to the variable response to clopidogrel is that clopidogrel is a prodrug requiring bioactivation to the active metabolite by hepatic cytochrome P450 enzymes (CYPs or P450s). P450s are inherently polymorphic and the activities of P450s are prone to induction and inhibition by numerous xenobiotics. Furthermore, extensive metabolism of clopidogrel in the liver primarily by P450s through multiple pathways leads to the formation of multiple metabolites, which significantly attenuate the formation of the active metabolite. These attrition pathways likely exacerbate the problems of the variable response. To overcome the interindividual variability, efforts have been made to mitigate the metabolic attritions as exemplified in the development of prasugrel, vicagrel, and reversible antithrombotic agents such as ticagrelor, cangrelor and elinogrel. The authors took a mechanistic approach to investigate the metabolism of clopidogrel by human liver microsomes (HLMs). The author's results demonstrated that formation of mixed disulfide conjugates between the active metabolite of clopidogrel and thiol reductants is an integral part of the bioactivation process in the liver. Furthermore, the authors found that mixed disulfide conjugates of clopidogrel are capable of releasing the active metabolite in the presence of glutathione without the need for P450-mediated bioactivation. Results from *ex vivo* studies using platelet-rich plasma revealed that these stable mixed disulfide conjugates of clopidogrel inhibit platelet aggregation when induced by adenosine diphosphate (ADP) agonist. Inhibition of platelet aggregation without the requirement of bioactivation by P450s holds great promise to overcome the interindividual variability in clopidogrel therapy.

Chapter 5 - Clopidogrel, is a cornerstone of therapy for acute coronary syndromes and the prevention of stent thrombosis after percutaneous coronary intervention. Hypersensitivity reactions to clopidogrel typically develop during the initial weeks of therapy and are severe enough to prompt drug discontinuation in 1 to 2% of patients. However, discontinuation of clopidogrel soon after percutaneous coronary intervention is problematic due to the risk of stent thrombosis. Accordingly, the management of clopidogrel hypersensitivity is of significant clinical importance. Clopidogrel desensitization protocols have been developed with success rates of at least 90%. These conventional desensitization methods require a washout period off of medication to allow the hypersensitivity symptoms to resolve before initiating desensitization. This strategy is undesirable in patients with coronary stents who are at risk for stent thrombosis if clopidogrel is withheld. Recent novel approaches have been described to treat clopidogrel hypersensitivity without drug interruption. Short-term corticosteroids and/or antihistamines are administered to suppress the hypersensitivity symptoms while facilitating the development of physiologic tolerance as clopidogrel is continued. Even after the antiallergy medications are terminated, successful desensitization is maintained during long-term therapy. Alternative antiplatelet drugs have recently become available but the safety and efficacy of these newer agents as potential substitute therapy for patients with clopidogrel hypersensitivity is yet to be determined.

Chapter 6 - Proton pump inhibitors often are prescribed in combination with clopidogrel to decrease the risk of gastrointestinal bleeding after an acute coronary syndrome. Clopidogrel is a prodrug that has to be metabolized in the liver to generate the active metabolite. Both medications are metabolized largely by the CYP2C19 enzyme, therefore concerns exist that a drug–drug interaction during concomitant treatment may result in a reduction of platelet inhibition. The authors have reviewed the observational and randomized control studies that have evaluated the potential influence of proton pump inhibitors on the inhibitory effect of clopidogrel, along with cardiovascular outcomes. The authors summarized regulatory and academic guidelines for treatment of patients in which concomitant therapy with clopidogrel and proton pump inhibitors may be indicated. Lastly the authors discuss confounding issues such as the differential effects of individual proton pump inhibitors on the pharmacodynamics of clopidogrel and variation in clopidogrel metabolism mediated by genetic polymorphisms of the CYP2C19 isoenzyme.

Chapter 7 - *Introduction:* There has been a significant increase in the volume of urological patients on daily clopidogrel therapy that require invasive elective urological procedures. In the present chapter the authors sought to assess current scientific evidence for appropriately managing this patient cohort during the perioperative period.

Methods: A literature search for English language publications using the PubMed® and Embase® databases was performed. Keywords included "clopidogrel," "perioperative management" and "urological surgery." A total of 148 articles were analysed, of which 86 were suitable for analysis based on clinical relevance and importance of content.

Results: Clopidogrel is compulsory for 4-6 weeks after insertion of bare metal stents (BMS). It is also mandatory for up to 12 months after insertion of drug-eluting stents (DES). Elective urological surgery must be either delayed beyond these waiting periods or performed with patients receiving daily clopidogrel as withdrawal of the agent results in a five- to ten-fold increase in the risk of postoperative MI, stent thrombosis or death. The risk of perioperative surgical bleeding is increased by 50% in patients where clopidogrel is continued.

Conclusion: The risk of cardiovascular morbidity (i.e. coronary thrombosis) when clopidogrel is discontinued before elective urological surgery is generally higher than the risk of perioperative bleeding when the agent is continued. It is imperative that urologists are familiar with standardised guidelines if this increasing patient cohort is to receive optimal perioperative management.

Chapter 8 - Dual oral antiplatelet therapy with aspirin and clopidogrel is the cornerstone of current therapy in patients with acute coronary syndromes and in patients undergoing percutaneous coronary intervention (PCI). Responsiveness to clopidogrel is not uniform and is subject to considerable interindividual variability. Furthermore, there are recent data that poor response to clopidogrel, or "high on-treatment platelet reactivity" (HPR), may be associated with the occurrence of ischemic events post-PCI. A variety of platelet function testing methods are currently available for evaluating platelet inhibition to clopidogrel, particularly in post-PCI patients, in order to determine and potentially reduce the individual risk for ischemic events. Platelet function testing offers the potential to individually tailor antiplatelet therapy.

Whether a personalized approach to intensified platelet inhibition therapy can be beneficial in higher risk patients remains to be determined and will require further prospective investigation. The authors will review in this chapter the impact of clopidogrel responsiveness on clinical outcomes and personalized antiplatelet strategies to improve clopidogrel responsiveness.

In: Clopidogrel
Editors: J. P. Alesci and A. Victorino
ISBN: 978-1-62948-336-8
© 2014 Nova Science Publishers, Inc.

Chapter 1

Clinical Review: Pharmacology of Traditional and Modern Anticoagulant and Antiplatelet Therapy

***Parth J. Parekh*[1], *Jonathan Merrell*[2], *John E. Brush*[3] *and David A. Johnson*[4]**

[1]Department of Internal Medicine, Eastern Virginia Medical School, Norfolk, VA, US

[2]Department of Pediatrics, Indiana University, Indianapolis, IN, US

[3]Sentara Cardiology Specialists, Norfolk, VA, US

[4]Department of Internal Medicine, Division of Gastroenterology, Eastern Virginia Medical School, Norfolk, VA, US

Abstract

Warfarin was the mainstay of oral anticoagulant therapy until the recent discovery of more precise targets for therapy. Although warfarin therapy is plagued by a narrow therapeutic index, variable individual metabolic responses, and numerous food and drug interactions, newer agents purport to rise above these setbacks. Furthermore, while the safety of these new drugs compared to traditional therapy has been called into question, [1] their ease of use makes it unlikely that they will disappear.

This review will explore the mechanisms of action and pharmacokinetics of traditional and novel anticoagulants and antiplatelet agents. In addition, recommended withholding periods for these drugs for patients undergoing elective endoscopic procedures as well as options for achieving rapid hemostasis in patients undergoing emergent endoscopy.

INTRODUCTION

The discovery of warfarin in the 1950s was a milestone in the development in anticoagulation. Warfarin was the first step towards using oral anticoagulants and it gave patients a viable alternative to heparin. Since the discovery of warfarin, however, there has been a large gap in the development of these drugs. Knowledge of the limitations in using warfarin including its narrow therapeutic index, numerous drug and food interactions, and its individual response variations has led to the development of new forms of anticoagulation. These newer agents target factor Xa, thrombin, and platelets both directly and indirectly to offer a safer and more effective alternative to warfarin. The rapidly growing list of these drugs, however, presents a challenge to endoscopists who must treat patients on these sundry medications. Understanding each drug and particularly understanding the necessary "washout" time for each prior to a procedure is vital and sadly missing in todays practice. This review is intended to summarize the pharmacologic highlights of traditional and modern anticoagulants and antiplatelet agents with particular attention to suggested “best practice” recommendations for the withholding of these drugs prior to endoscopic procedures.

THE COAGULATION PATHWAY

Endothelium–platelet interactions and the coagulation cascade serve as the focal points of hemostasis. In primary hemostasis, the endothelium of a damaged vessel releases adenosine diphosphate (ADP), serotonin, and thromboxane A2. Platelets respond to these cytokines with expression of glycoprotein IIb/IIIa and platelet-endothelial cell adhesion molecule 1 (PECAM1) to form an initial platelet plug. [2] The coagulation cascade unfolds simultaneously with its intrinsic and extrinsic pathways that lead to the formation of fibrin. [3] Figure 1 below depicts both the intrinsic and extrinsic pathways that comprise the coagulation cascade.

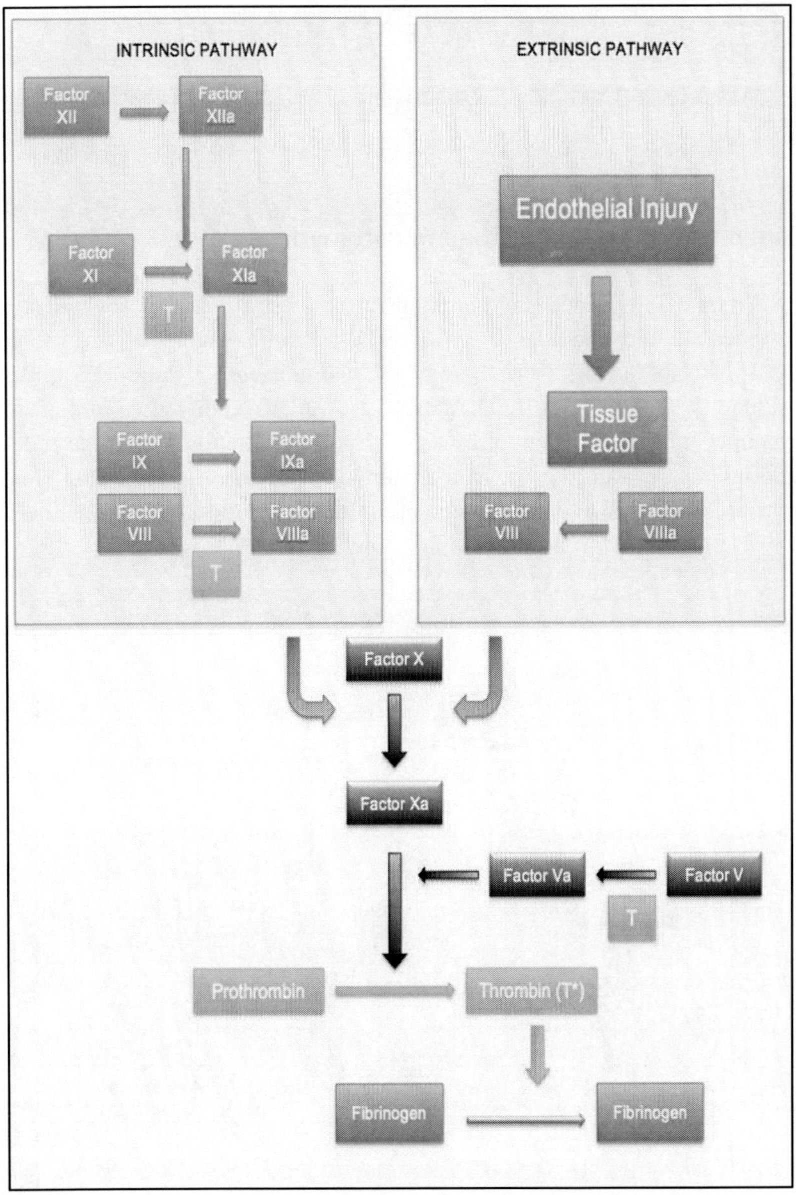

Figure 1. The intrinsic and extrinsic pathways of coagulation the coagulation cascade. [81]

VITAMIN K ANTAGONISTS

Warfarin (Coumadin®, Jantoven®, Marevan®, Lawarin®, Waran®, Warfant®)

Pharmacokinetics and Pharmacodynamics

Vitamin K is a necessary participant in the synthesis of several proteins that mediate the coagulation cascade. Warfarin antagonizes the effects of vitamin K and as a result inhibits the gamma carboxylation of glutamate residues in factors II, VII, IX and X as well as endogenous anticoagulant proteins C and S. In addition, warfarin inhibits vitamin K epoxide reductase subsequently preventing the conversion of vitamin K 2,3-epoxide (inactive form) to vitamin K hydroquinone (active form). [4] Figure 2 depicts the effect of warfarin on the formation of a thrombus.

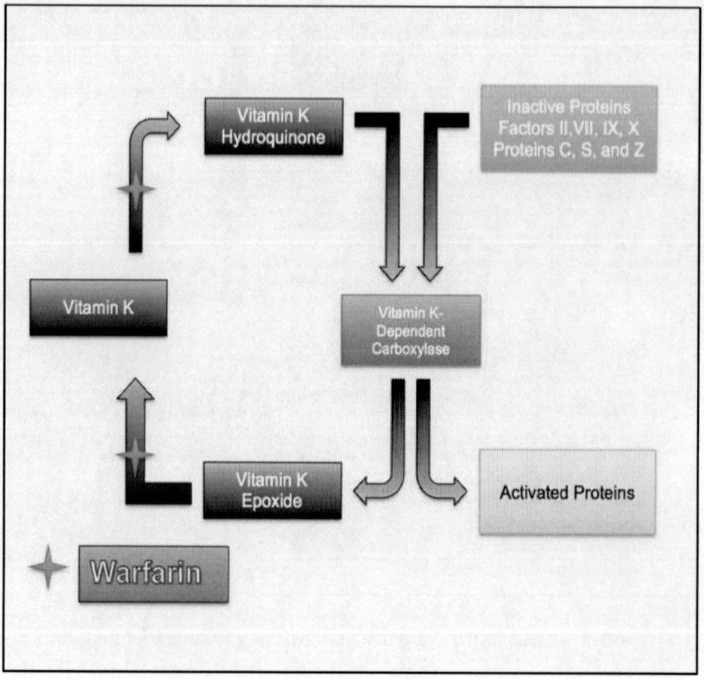

Figure 2. The mechanism of action of warfarin. [82]

Warfarin is indicated for the treatment of venous thrombosis and pulmonary embolism, prophylaxis and treatment of thromboembolic complications associated with atrial fibrillation and/or cardiac valve replacement, and the reduction in the risk of death, recurrent myocardial infarction and thromboembolic events, i.e. stroke or systemic embolization, after a myocardial infarction. Dosed as a once daily oral tablet, warfarin attains a peak concentration 72-96 hours after dosage with a half-life of 20-60 hours (mean of 40 hours). Warfarin is eliminated entirely by metabolism, namely the cytochrome P-450 (CYP450) enzyme that metabolizes warfarin to its inactive metabolites therefore special consideration should be given to medications co-administered with warfarin. [5]

Adverse Effects

Side effects of warfarin include bleeding (particularly if used in conjunction with other anticoagulants), necrosis of skin and other tissues (i.e. purple toe syndrome), systemic atheroemboli and cholesterol microemboli, anaphylaxis, vasculitis, elevated transaminases, cholestatic hepatitis (when used in conjunction with ticlopidine), nausea, vomiting, diarrhea, abdominal pain, flatulence, rash, dermatitis, tracheal or tracheobronchial calcifications. [4]

Prior to initiating or while on warfarin therapy close scrutiny should be given to any medications or herbal supplements patients may be taking in addition to warfarin. The cytochrome P-450 enzyme responsible for metabolism of warfarin to its inactive metabolites is affected by a myriad of agents. [4] Drug-drug interactions include metronidazole, cephalosporins and fluconazole, in addition to any agent that may enhance or inhibit the CYP450 pathway (see Table 1 below for full list). Dietary restrictions also have to be considered as foods rich in vitamin K (spinach, collard greens, beets) may also alter warfarin levels. It should also be noted that when warfarin is administered to patients with myocardial infarction, the essential oil of garlic increased fibrinolysis by 63% to 69% thereby enhancing the activity of warfarin. [6]

Table 1. Medications affecting the CYP pathway [83]

Enzyme	Inhibitors	Inducers
CYP2C9	amiodarone, capecitabine, cotrimoxazole, etravirine, fluconazole, fluvastatin, fluvoxamine, metronidazole, miconazole, oxandrolone, sulfinpyrazone, tigecycline, voriconazole, zafirlukast	aprepitant, bosentan, carbamazepine, phenobarbital, rifampin
CYP1A2	acyclovir, allopurinol, caffeine, cimetidine, ciprofloxacin, disulfiram, enoxacin, famotidine, fluvoxamine, methoxsalen, mexiletine, norfloxacin, oral contraceptives, phenylpropanolamine, propafenone, propranolol, terbinafine, thiabendazole, ticlopidine, verapamil, zileuton	montelukast, moricizine, omeprazole, phenobarbital, phenytoin, cigarette smoke
CYP3A4	alprazolam, amiodarone, amlodipine, amprenavir, aprepitant, atorvastatin, atazanavir, biclutamide, ciostazol, cimetidine, ciprofloxacin, clarithromycin, conivaptan, cyclosporine, darunavir/ritonavir, diltiazem, erythromycin, fluconazole, fluoxetine, fluvoxamine, fosamprenavir, imatinib, indinavir, isoniazid, itraconazole, ketoconazole, lopinavir/ritonavir, nefazodone, nelfinavir, nilotinib, oral contraceptives, posaconazole, ranitidine, ranolazine, ritonavir, saquinavir, telithromycin, tipranavir, voriconazole, zileuton	armodafinil, amprenavir, aprepitant, bosentan, carbamazepine, efavirenz, entravirine, modafinil, nafcillin, phenytoin, pioglitazone, prednisone, rifampin, rufinamide

Reversal Agents

Fresh frozen plasma and vitamin K remains the mainstay in warfarin reversal. Table 2 below outlines the protocol of reversing warfarin in the event of an acute bleed or supra-therapeutic INR in the absence of bleeding.

Monitoring

There are several variables that ought to be taken into consideration prior to initiating warfarin and maintaining a therapeutic INR. The guidelines outlined in Table 3 are a level 1 recommendation for the initiation and monitoring of warfarin therapy. Current recommendations include checking an INR at least 4 times during the first week of therapy, using lower initial dosages in those above the age of 75 or a weight of less than 60 kg and higher initial dosages in younger patients or if the patient is on medications known to lower the effects of warfarin or a diet rich in vitamin K. [7]

Table 2. Management of supra-therapeutic INR [84]

Clinical Scenario	Intervention
INR > Therapeutic Range but < 5.0; Bleeding Absent	• Lower the dose or withhold next dose; Resume at a lower dose when INR approaches therapeutic range • If INR only minimally above therapeutic range (up to 10%) dose reduction may not be necessary
INR 5.0 – 9.0; Bleeding Absent (Risk increases exponentially from an INR of 5.0-9.0)	• Withhold warfarin therapy • If high risk of bleeding, administer vitamin K (1.0-2.0 mg PO or 0.5-1.0 mg IV) • Measure INR within 24 hours; reduce warfarin at a reduced dose when INR is in therapeutic range
INR > 9.0; Bleeding Absent	• If low risk of bleeding, cease warfarin therapy and administer vitamin K (2.5-5.0 mg PO or 1.0 mg IV). Measure INR within 6-12 hours; resume warfarin at a reduced dose when INR is in therapeutic range • If high risk of bleeding, cease warfarin therapy and administer vitamin K (1.0 mg IV). Consider Prothrombinex- HT (25-50 IU/kg) and fresh frozen plasma (FFP) (150-300 mL), measure INR in 6-12 hours; resume warfarin at a reduced dose when INR is in therapeutic range
Clinically Significant Bleeding	• Cease warfarin therapy, give 5.0-10.0 mg vitamin K IV as well as Prothrombinex- HT (25-50 IU/kg) and FFP (150-300 mL); Assess patient continuously until INR < 5.0 and bleeding stops. OR • If FFP unavailable cease warfarin therapy and administer vitamin K (5.0-10.0 mg IV) and Prothrombinex- HT (25-50 IU/kg); Assess patient continuously until INR < 5.0 and bleeding stops. OR • If Prothrombinex- HT unavailable cease warfarin therapy and administer vitamin K (5.0-10.0 mg IV) and FFP (10-15 mL/kg); Assess patient continuously until INR < 5.0 and bleeding stops.
Bleeding Risks	• High – active gastrointestinal disorders (inflammatory bowel disease or peptic ulcer disease); patients receiving concomitant antiplatelet therapy; patients with thrombocytopenia; those who underwent a major surgical procedure within the preceding two weeks

When heparin is used concomitantly as a bridge to warfarin, special considerations should be taken. It is recommended to overlap warfarin therapy for 4-5 days until warfarin has produced the desired therapeutic response. The INR should be monitored at least 5 hours after the last intravenous bolus dose of heparin, 4 hours after cessation of a continuous intravenous infusion of heparin or 24 hours after the last subcutaneous injection of heparin. [4]

Table 3. Initiation and monitoring of warfarin therapy [85]

		5 mg Initiation	10 mg Initiation
Day	INR	Dose	Dose
1	-	5 mg	10 mg
2	<1.5	5 mg	7.5-10 mg
	1.5-1.9	2.5 mg	2.5 mg
	2.0-2.5	1-2.5 mg	1-2.5 mg
	>2.5	0	0
3	<1.5	5-10 mg	5-10 mg
	1.5-1.9	2.5-5 mg	2.5-5 mg
	2.0-2.5	0-2.5 mg	0-2.5 mg
	2.5-3	0-2.5 mg	0-2.5 mg
	>3	0	0
4	<1.5	10 mg	10 mg
	1.5-1.9	5-7.5 mg	5 – 7.5 mg
	2.0-3.0	0-5 mg	0-5 mg
	>3	0	0
5	<1.5	10 mg	10 mg
	1.5-1.9	7.5-10 mg	7.5-10 mg
	2.0-3.0	0-5 mg	0-5 mg
	>3	0	0
6	<1.5	7.5-12.5 mg	7.5-12.5 mg
	1.5-1.9	5-10 mg	5-10 mg
	2.0-3.0	0-7.5 mg	0-7.5 mg
	>3	0	0

Recommended Withholding Period Prior to Endoscopic Procedures

If the annual risk for thromboembolism is low, warfarin should be discontinued 4-5 days prior to a procedure. Patients with prosthetic heart valves, however, have an increased risk for thromboembolism and careful consideration should be given to the perioperative management of their anticoagulation. Although there are no formal guidelines regarding optimal management, some prospective studies have shown a 1% risk of experiencing a thromboembolic event for patients on long-term warfarin therapy undergoing minor invasive procedures that have been taken off oral anticoagulation for up to 5 days prior. [8]

Xa Inhibitors

The factor Xa inhibitors competitively inhibit activated factor X. Factor Xa unifies the intrinsic and extrinsic pathways, therefore these drugs impact the coagulation cascade as a whole. Normally, factor Xa forms a complex with factor Va called prothrombinase. [9] This enzyme complex then cleaves prothrombin to form the active agent, thrombin (see Figure 3). Factor Xa inhibitors bind to the active site of factor Xa preventing the formation of prothrombinase. [10]

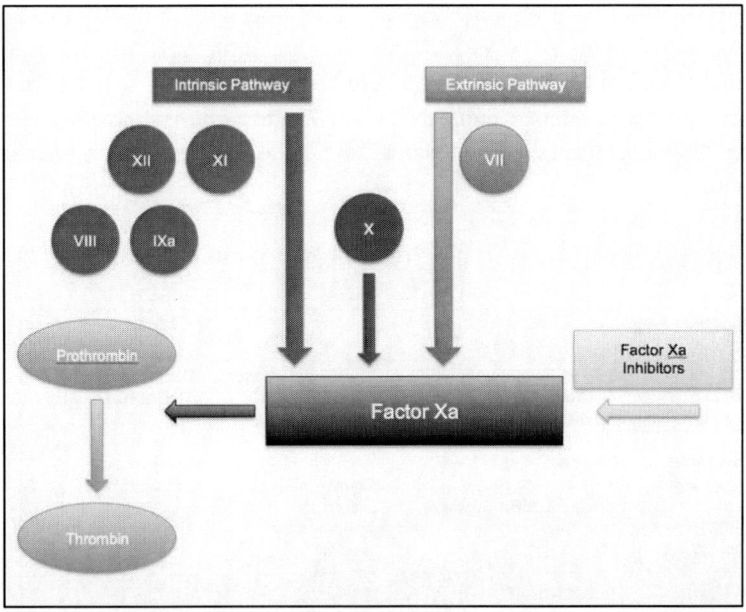

Figure 3. Mechanism of action of Xa inhibitors. [86]

Rivaroxaban (Xarelto®)

Rivaroxaban is a direct factor Xa inhibitor approved for use in nonvalvular atrial fibrillation and DVT and PE treatment and prophylaxis following large joint replacement. [11]

Pharmacokinetics and Pharmacodynamics

Dosed as a once daily or twice daily oral tablet, rivaroxaban attains a peak concentration 2.5-4 hours after dosage with a half-life of 5-9 hours (9-13 in elderly). [12] Current manufacturer recommendations are to use with caution in patients with moderate renal impairment (defined as a CrCl 30 to 50mL/min) and to avoid in patients with severe renal impairment (defined as CrCl <30mL/min). Regarding hepatic function, there was a noted increase in exposure to rivaroxaban when observed in patients with moderate hepatic impairment (Child-Pugh class B) however there are currently no recommendations on dose adjustment based on hepatic function. [11,12] The drug is a substrate of CYP3A4 and P-glycoprotein (P-gp) transporters. Therefore special consideration should be given when co-administering medications that inhibit or induce the CYP450 enzymes (see Table 1 for full list) or P-gp transport (see Table 4 for full list) as this may change riraoxaban exposure. [13]

Table 4. Medications requiring P-glycoprotein transporters [87]

Substrates			Inhibitors
Antacids	**β-Adrenoceptor antagonist**	**Immunosuppressants**	**Diverse Inhibitors**
Cimetidine	Bunitrolol	Cyclosporine A	Verapamil
Ranitidine	Carvedilol	Sirolimus	Quinidine
	Tanilol	Tacrolimus	Valspodar
Antibiotics	Reserpine		Cyclosporine
Erythromycin		**Opioids**	Ketoconazole
Tetracycline	**Calcium Channel Blockers**	Loperamide	
Rifampin	Diltiazem	Domperidone	
Levofloxacin	Mibefradil	Morphine	
		Pentazocine	
Antiemetic	**Antiarrhythmic**	Methadone	
Odansetron	Dignoxin	Asimadoline	
		Fentanyl	
Chemotherapy	**H1 Antagonists**		
Paclitaxel	Fexofenadine	**Steroids**	
Doxorubicin	Terfenadine	Dexamethasone	
Daunorubicin		Methylprednisolone	
Vinblastine	**HIV Protease Inhibitors**	Aldosterone	
Vincristine	Amprenavir	Progesterone	
Actinomycin D	Indinavir	Hydrocortisone	
Docetaxel	Nelfinavir	Cortisol	
Etoposide	Saquinavir	Corticosterone	
Imatinib	Ritonavir		
Teniposide		**Others**	
		Colchicine	
		Itraconazole	
		Phenothiazines	
		Ivermectin	

Adverse Effects

Adverse effects of rivaroxaban include bleeding, agranulocytosis, jaundice, cholestasis, hepatitis, and hypersensitivity reactions. [11]

Reversal Agents

There are currently no reversal agents that can be used in the event of an acute bleed in patients on rivaroxaban. Current recommendations are the use of recombinant activated factor VII (rfVIIa) and prothrombin complex concentrate (PCC). [14]

Recommended Withholding Period Prior to Endoscopic Procedures

Rivaroxaban should be discontinued at least 24 hours prior to any procedure in individuals with normal kidney function. An extended washout time of 48 hours is recommended for patients with a CrCl <50mL/min and elderly patients in general. [15,16]

Apixaban (Eliquis®)

The results of the ARISTOTLE trial led the FDA announced its approval for apixiban for the prevention of stroke and thromboembolism in patients with nonvalvular atrial fibrillation on December 28th, 2012. [17] Agnelli et al published results from the AMPLIFY trial, a double-blinded study in which 2482 patients received either 2.5mg or 5mg apixaban BID for one year for extended treatment of venous thromboembolisms. Those treated with 2.5mg apixaban BID were found to experience 7.2% fewer thromboembolic events than patients treated with placebo (95% confidence interval, 5.0 to 9.3). While those treated with 5mg apixaban BID experienced 7.0% fewer thromboembolic than those treated with placebo (95% confidence interval, 4.0 to 9.1). [18]Apixaban is currently under review by the FDA for approval for its use in DVT prophylaxis following large joint surgery.

Pharmacokinetics and Pharmacodynamics

Apixaban's mechanism of action is identical to that of rivaroxaban. Dosed as a twice-daily oral tablet, apixaban attains a peak concentration 1-3 hours after dosage with a half-life of 8-13 hours. The drug relies primarily on the CYP3A4 system for full metabolism therefore potent CYP inducers or inhibitors as seen in Table 1 should be discontinued 14 days prior to initiation of apixaban therapy and avoided while on therapy.[19]

Adverse Effects

Common adverse effects of apixaban (seen in 1 to 10 out of 100 patients) include bleeding, anemia, easy bruising, and nausea. [19]

Reversal Agents

There are currently no reversal agents that can be used in the event of an acute bleed in patients on apixaban. Current recommendations are the use of recombinant activated factor VII (rfVIIa) and prothrombin complex concentrate (PCC). [19]

Recommended Withholding Period Prior to Endoscopic Procedures

Apixiaban should be discontinued at least 24 hours before any elective procedure with a low risk of bleeding, particularly in a location that would be noncritical and easily controlled. In anticipation of an invasive procedure with a moderate or high risk of clinically significant bleeding, Apixaban should be discontinued at least 48 hours prior to the procedure. [20]

Direct Thrombin Inhibitors

The direct thrombin inhibitors (DTIs) directly inhibit the enzyme thrombin. DTI's are divided into two classes: the bivalents, which bind to both the thrombin active site and exosite-1, and the univalents, which bind solely to the active site. [21] Figure 4 depicts the effect of DTIs on thrombin.

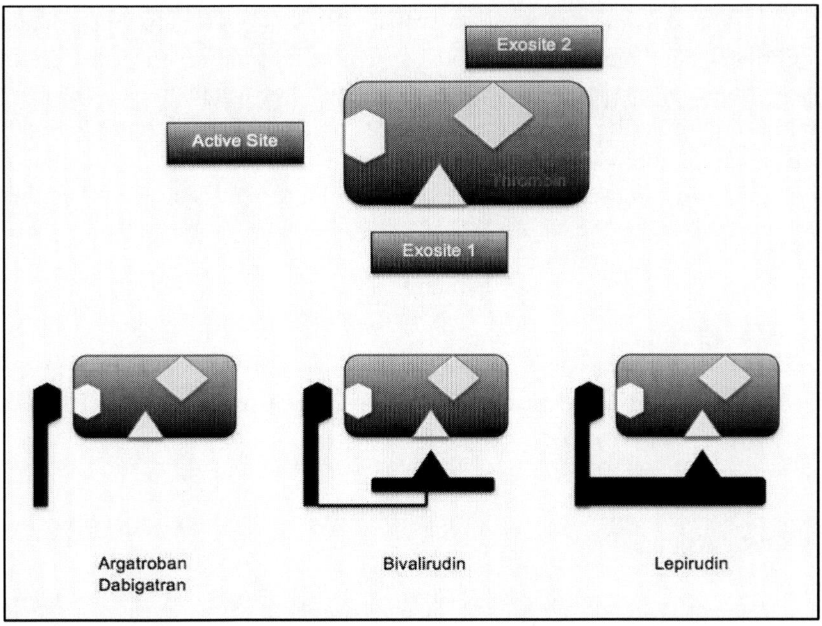

Figure 4. Mechanism of action of univalent and bivalent DTIs. [88]

Lepirudin (Refludan®)

The bivalent DTIs were discovered because of *Hirudo Medicinalis,* the medicinal leech.[22] Leech saliva contains an anticoagulant agent, which was subsequently isolated and modified to produce the modern bivalent DTIs. Lepirudin is a member of the bivalent class of DTIs. Lepirudin itself is a recombinant hirudin derived from yeast cells, which is a highly specific inhibitor of thrombin. It is commonly used in patients with heparin-induced thrombocytopenia who require ongoing anticoagulation. [23]

Pharmacokinetics and Pharmacodynamics

Lepirudin irreversibly binds to free and clot-bound thrombin thus inhibiting the activation of factors V, VIII, XIII, and conversion of fibrinogen to fibrin. Administered intravenously, lepirudin achieves a peak plasma concentration in approximately 10 minutes and has a half-life of 1.3 hours. Renal excretion is the predominant elimination pathway with more than 80% of available lepirudin eliminated unchanged. Thus particular attention should be given to ensuring sufficient kidney function in patients started on lepirudin. [24]

Adverse Effects

Adverse effects of lepirudin include excessive bleeding and potentially severe hypersensitivity reactions. [24]

Reversal Agents

There are currently no reversal agents available in the event of an acute bleed in patients on lepirudin. [24] Blood products such as fresh frozen plasma remain the mainstay of treatment in case of bleeding. Hemodialysis appears ineffective in rapidly lowering the plasma concentration of lepirudin. [24] In contrast, plasmapheresis with fine filters (pore size of 15000 Da) has been shown to rapidly remove hirudin, another bivalent direct thrombin inhibitor, from the blood and may be considered for reversal of lepirudin. [26]

Recommended Withholding Period Prior to Endoscopic Procedures

There is limited data available on the optimum withholding period prior to endoscopic procedures pertaining to patients on lepirudin. The current recommendations are to obtain an aPTT to confirm a return to normal hemostasis prior to undergoing procedures. [27]

BIVALIRUDIN (ANGIOMAX®)

Bivalirudin is a synthetic peptide analog of hirudin and a bivalent DTI. It is approved for use in patients undergoing percutaneous coronary intervention (PCI) with provisional use of glycoprotein IIb/IIIa inhibitors, patients with or at risk of heparin-induced thrombocytopenia or in patients with unstable angina undergoing percutaneous transluminal coronary angioplasty. [28] The American College of Chest Physicians (ACCP) advocates the use of bivalirudin in combination with clopidogrel as opposed to heparin for initial antithrombotic therapy in patients at moderate to high risk for an ischemic event and who are scheduled for very early coronary angiography (within <6 hours). [29] The HORIZONS-AMI Trial randomized 3,602 patients with ST-segment elevation myocardial infarction (STEMI) who presented within 12 hours of onset of symptoms and subsequently undergoing primary PCI to anticoagulation with bivalirudin alone or heparin plus a glycoprotein IIb/IIIa inhibitor. Stone et al concluded that in patients with STEMI who are undergoing primary PCI, anticoagulation with bivalirudin alone results in significantly reduced 30-day rates of major bleeding and net adverse clinical events as compared to heparin plus glycoprotein IIb/IIIa inhibitors. [30]

Pharmacokinetics and Pharmacodynamics

Bivalirudin is a reversible direct thrombin inhibitor that binds to circulating and clot-bound thrombin. The inhibition of thrombin prevents various steps in the coagulation process, such as the activation of factors V, VIII, XIII, the conversion of fibrinogen to fibrin, and platelet activation and aggregation. [31]

Administered intravenously, bivalirudin achieves an immediate peak plasma concentration with a half-life of 22 minutes. Approximately 20% of unchanged bivalirudin is renally excreted, and the remainder undergoes intracellular proteolysis. Thus particular consideration should be given to patients with severe renal impairment or in dialysis-dependent patients. Current recommendations are to adjust the dose for renal impairment in patients with a CrCL of 10-29mL/min undergoing PCI and in patients with a CrCl <60mL/min being treated for heparin induced thrombocytopenia. Current manufacturer recommendations state that dosing modifications are not necessary in patients with hepatic impairment. [28]

Adverse Effects

Adverse effects of bivalirudin include excessive bleeding, back pain, nausea, hypotension, bradycardia and headache. [28]

Reversal Agents

There are presently no reversal agents that can be used in the event of an acute bleed in patients on bivalirudin. Current guidelines suggest that modified ultrafiltration and hemodialysis may facilitate the removal of bivalirudin with modified ultrafiltration (removal of between 45-69% depending on filter type) being superior to hemodialysis (removal of 25%). Recombinant factor VII (rFVIIa) has can be administered at a dose of 90 mcg/kg. Lastly, blood products such as fresh frozen plasma or cryoprecipitate can be given to work as a competitor to displace bivalirudin from thrombin. [32,33]

Recommended Withholding Period Prior to Endoscopic Procedures

Due to its short half-life, an infusion of bivalirudin need only be discontinued prior to induction of anesthesia in a patient with normal renal function. [34]

DABIGATRAN (PRADAXA®)

Dabigatran is a monovalent DTI that is currently approved for the prevention of stroke in non-valvular atrial fibrillation. [35] Schulman et al. recently found dabigatran to be effective in the extended treatment of venous thromboembolism. There was a lower risk of major or clinically relevant bleeding when compared to warfarin but a higher risk than placebo. [36]

Pharmacokinetics and Pharmacodynamics

Dabigatran competitively binds to free and clot-bound thrombin thus preventing the activation of fibrinogen, clotting cofactors, and the eventual formation of a clot. Dosed as a twice-daily oral tablet, dabigatran reaches a peak plasma concentration after 1-2 hours with a half-life of 12-17 hours. Renal clearance accounts for 80-85% elimination of dabigatran. Doses should be reduced in patients with moderate renal impairment (defined as CrCl 30-50 mL/min) and should be avoided in patients with severe renal impairment (defined CrCl 15-30 mL/min) and concomitant use of medications requiring use of P-glycoprotein (see Table 2). Current manufacturer recommendations state that dosing modifications are not necessary in patients with hepatic impairment. [37]

Adverse Effects

Adverse effects of dabigatran include bleeding and GI irritation such as GERD, esophagitis and erosive gastritis. [38]

Reversal Agents

To date, there are no available antidotes for dabigatran. Blood products, such as fresh frozen plasma, are the principal agents of reversal. Hemodialysis may be effective in removing as much as 60% of circulating drug since the majority of dabigtran is unbound to protein, however there is insufficient data to support this as a means of a reversal. [39,40]

Recommended Withholding Period Prior to Endoscopic Procedures

For patients with normal renal function and high risk of bleeding or major surgery, it is recommended to withhold for 2 days, and for otherwise average risks, for 24 hours. [35] Table 5 illustrates manufacturer recommendations for the discontinuation of dabigatran prior to elective surgery, as stratified by renal function.

Table 5. Manufacturer Recommendations for Discontinuation of Dabigatran Prior to Elective Surgery [35]

Renal Function (CrCL* mL/min)	Mean Half-life (Hours)	Standard Risk of Bleeding	High Risk of Bleeding
>80	13 (11-22)	24 Hours	2-4 Days
50-80	15 (12-34)	24 Hours	2-4 Days
30-50	18 (13-23)	>48 Hours	>4 Days
<30	27 (22-35)	48-120 Hours	>5 Days

* Creatinine Clearance.

ADP ANTAGONISTS (THIENOPYRIDINES)

During primary hemostasis, damaged endothelium release ADP causing the recruitment and activation of platelets. This aggregation leads to the formation of the primary platelet plug, which must be stabilized, by the formation of fibrin. [41] The thienopyridines block the ADP-dependent aggregation of platelets by inhibiting the $P2Y_{12}$ receptor. Figure 5 depicts the effect of thienopyridines on platelet aggregation.

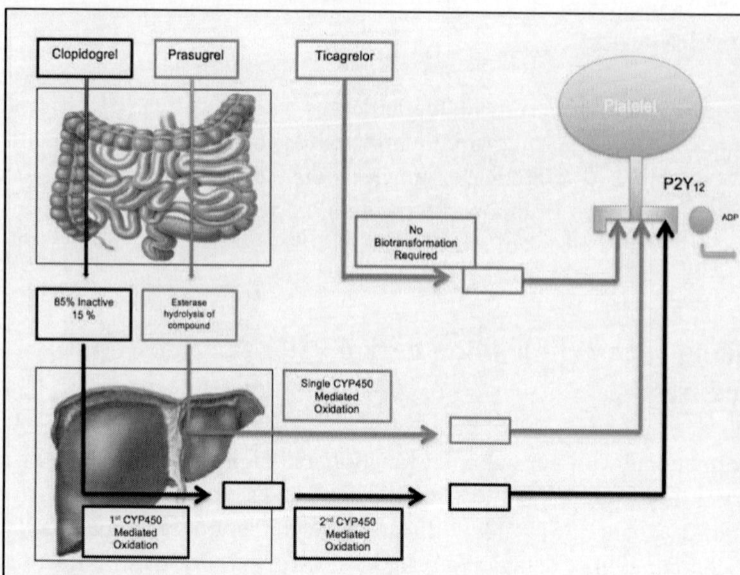

Figure 5. Mechanism of action of thienopyridines on platelet aggregation. [89]

TICLOPIDINE (TICLID®)

Ticlopidine is a thienopyridine approved for its use in patients for the prevention of thromboembolic stroke, acute coronary syndrome, and for post coronary stent placement to prevent stent thrombosis. [42]

Pharmacokinetics and Pharmacodynamics

Ticlopidine is a pro-drug that is metabolized to its active form in the liver. The active metabolite then irreversibly inhibits ADP-induced platelet-fibrinogen binding and subsequent platelet-platelet interactions. Dosed as a twice-daily oral tablet, ticlopidine reaches its peak plasma concentration in 2 hours with a half-life of 12 hours. It is metabolized in the liver and is primarily eliminated via renal excretion therefore particular consideration should be given to those with renal or hepatic impairment. [43,44]

Adverse Effects

Ticlopidine is known for its steep side-effect profile, which includes neutropenia, thrombocytopenia, agranulocytosis, thrombotic thrombocytepenic purpura (TTP), and aplastic anemia. [44]

Reversal Agents

There are currently no reversal agents that can be used in the event of an acute bleed in patients on ticlopidine. Current protocols for reversal in the setting of an acute bleed include 1 unit of platelet apheresis. When TTP is of concern, however, platelet apheresis should be avoided as this may accelerate thrombosis. [44]

Monitoring

Complete blood counts and leukocyte differentials should be performed prior to initiation of therapy and every 2 weeks to the end of the third month of therapy. Continue monitoring for at least two weeks following discontinuance of ticlopidine within the first 3 months of therapy. [44]

Recommended Withholding Period Prior to Endoscopic Procedures

Ticlopidine should be discontinued at least 7-10 days prior to any procedure, with consideration of up 10-14 days for procedures with a high propensity of bleeding. [34]

Clopidogrel (Plavix®)

Clopidogrel is a thienopyridine approved for use in patients with acute coronary syndrome who are managed medically or with coronary revascularization. In addition, clopidogrel is indicated following myocardial infarction, stroke, or established peripheral arterial disease to reduce the risk of new myocardial infarction, ischemic stroke, and other vascular death. [45]

Pharmacokinetics and Pharmacodynamics

Clopidogrel is a pro-drug which the CYP450 enzyme must metabolize in order to produce its active metabolite. The active metabolite then irreversibly inhibits the $P2Y_{12}$ substrate, which is necessary in the activation of platelets and eventual fibrin cross-linking. Ultimately, this inhibits platelet aggregation via the glycoprotein IIb/IIIa pathway. [45]

Dosed as a once daily oral tablet, clopidogrel attains peak plasma concentration 1 hour after dosage with a half-life of 7-8 hours. Clopidogrel and certain proton pump inhibitors are dependent on the CYP2C19 hepatic enzyme for their metabolism, because of this the FDA recommends against co-administration of clopidogrel and omeprazole or esomeprazole. [45] This interaction, however, has only been demonstrated in vitro and recent meta-analyses indicate that the clinical implications are insignificant. [46] There is limited data regarding the use of clopidogrel in renal or hepatic impairment therefore no dose adjustment is necessary in these populations. [45]

Adverse Effects

Adverse effects of clopidogrel include bleeding, thrombocytopenia, TTP, as well as GI disturbances including nausea, diarrhea or constipation. [45]

Reversal Agents

To date, there are no available reversal agents that can be used in the event of an acute bleed in patients on clopidogrel. Current guidelines state that blood products, such as fresh frozen plasma or cryoprecipitate are the primary agents of reversal. Several case reports have indicated potential reversal of Plavix with use of methylprednisolone and DDAVP. [45]

Recommended Withholding Period Prior to Endoscopic Procedures

Clopidogrel should be discontinued 5-7 days prior to any procedure where therapeutic intervention is anticipated or planned. [47]

Prasugrel (Effient®)

Prasugrel is a thienopyridine approved for the prevention of thrombotic cardiovascular events (including stent thrombosis) in patients with unstable angina, non-ST-elevation myocardial infarction or ST-elevation myocardial infarction who are to be managed with PCI. [48]

In 2007, Wivott et al presented the results of the TRITON-TIMI 38 trial, which was a head-to-head comparison of prasugrel versus clopidogrel in patients with acute coronary syndromes. 13,608 patients with moderate to high-risk coronary syndromes with scheduled PCI were randomized to receive prasugrel or clopidogrel. The authors concluded prasugrel to be associated with significantly reduced rates of ischemic events, including stent thrombosis, however there was an increased associated risk of major bleeding, including fatal bleeding in this patient population. Overall, there was no mortality benefit between the two groups. [49]

Pharmacokinetics and Pharmacodynamics

Prasugrel is a thienopyridine derivative that is structurally and pharmacologically related to clopidogrel, but exhibits more rapid, consistent, and greater inhibition of ADP-mediated platelet aggregation. Its increased potency appears to be a result of more efficient conversion of the pro-drug to its active metabolite. [50]

Dosed as a once daily oral tablet, prasugrel attains a peak plasma concentration 0.5 hours after dosage with a half-life of 2 to 15 hours. Prasugrel is metabolized principally by CYP3A4 and CYP2B6, and to a lesser extent by CYP2C9 and CYP2C19. Therefore, clinically significant interactions mediated by CYP enzymes are unlikely.[51] Prasugrel is primarily excreted in the urine as an inactive metabolite and thus particular attention should be paid to those with renal impairment. In patients with end-stage renal impairment, exposure to active metabolite was decreased to approximately half that in healthy individuals and those with moderate renal impairment. In low-weight individuals (weight <60 kg), increased exposure to the active metabolite is observed. [48]

Adverse Effects

Adverse effects of prasugrel includes bleeding, hypertension, hyperlipidemia, headache, backpain, anemia, and GI disturbances namely diarrhea. [48]

Reversal Agents

To date, there are no available reversal agents that can be used in the event of an acute bleed in patients on prasugrel. Current guidelines state that blood products, such as fresh frozen plasma or cryoprecipitate are the primary agents of reversal. [48]

Recommended Withholding Period Prior to Endoscopic Procedures

Prasugrel should be discontinued at least 7 days prior to any procedure where therapeutic intervention is anticipated or planned. [52]

TICAGRELOR (BRILLINTA®)

Ticagrelor is indicated for acute coronary syndrome, prevention of thrombotic events, and myocardial infarction with STEMI. [53]

In 2009, Wallentin et al presented the results of the PLATO trial, which was a head-to-head comparison of ticagrelor versus clopidogrel in patients with acute coronary syndromes. 18,624 patients with acute coronary syndrome, with or without ST-sgement elevation were randomized to receive ticarelor or clopidogrel. The authors concluded treatment with ticagrelor as compared with clopidogrel to be associated with reduced risk for stroke, myocardial infarction and death with no difference in rates of major bleeding. [54]

Pharmacokinetics and Pharmacodynamics

Ticagrelor differs from other thienopyridines in that it is a direct-acting $P2Y_{12}$ inhibitor, which changes conformation of the $P2Y_{12}$ receptor for reversible, concentration-dependent inhibition. Ticagrelor is metabolized to form an active metabolite, but the active metabolite has very similar pharmacokinetics to the parent compound. The drug does not necessarily require metabolic conversion to interact with the receptor, likely contributing to the drug's higher efficacy over clopidogrel. [55]

Dosed as a once or twice daily oral tablet, ticagrelor attains a peak plasma concentration of 1.5 hours after dosage with a half-life of 7-8.5 hours. The primary route of excretion is via hepatic metabolism thus precaution should be given to those with hepatic dysfunction. [52,53] Ticagrelor is dependent on the CYP3A3 enzyme for its metabolism, therefore inducers and inhibitors should be carefully considered prior to co-administration (see Table 1). Since ticagrelor does not require hepatic activation, it may be more effective for patients with CYP2C19 genetic variants than other drugs in its class. Current manufacturer recommendations state that dosing modifications are not necessary in patients with renal impairment and mild hepatic impairment. In patients with moderate hepatic impairment, current manufacturers recommend exercise caution as data is limited, and in patients with severe hepatic impairment ticagrelor is contraindicated. [53]

Adverse Effects

Adverse effects of ticagrelor include bleeding, dyspnea, headache, cough, and GI disturbances including nausea and diarrhea. [53]

Reversal Agents

To date, there are no available reversal agents that can be used in the event of an acute bleed in patients on direct thrombin inhibitors. Current guidelines state that blood products, such as fresh frozen plasma or cryoprecipitate are the primary agents of reversal. [53]

Recommended Withholding Period Prior to Endoscopic Procedures

Ticagrelor should be discontinued a minimum of 5 days prior to any procedure where therapeutic intervention is anticipated or planned. [56]

Glycoprotein IIB/IIIA Inhibitors

Glycoprotein IIb/IIIa antagonists inhibit glycoprotein IIb/IIIa (also referred to as integrin $\alpha_{IIb}\beta_3$), a complex of integrin found on platelets. The activation of the integrin complex enables the binding of fibrinogen, platelet-platelet adhesion, and endothelial adherence. Glycoprotein IIb/IIIa inhibitors act on this receptor. [57] Figure 6 depicts the effect of glycoprotein IIb/IIIa inhibitors on the formation of a platelet plug.

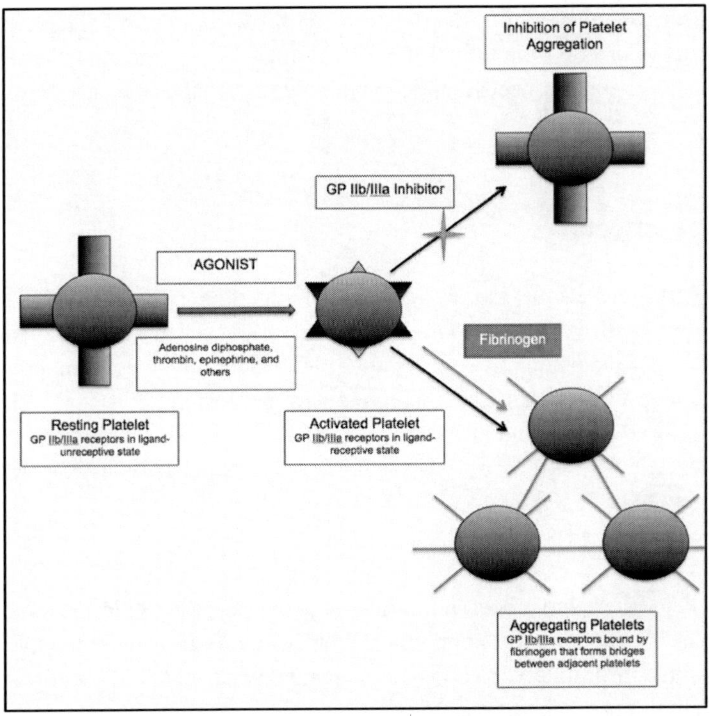

Figure 6.Mechanism of action of GP IIb/IIIa inhibitors. [90]

ABCIXIMAB (REOPRO®)

Abciximab is approved for its use in individuals undergoing PCI (with or without stent placement). [58]

Pharmacokinetics and Pharmacodynamics

Abciximab is a chimeric monoclonal antibody fab (fragment antigen binding) that inhibits platelet aggregation by binding to the GPIIb/IIIa receptor. Abciximab is dosed as an intravenous bolus administered 10-60 minutes prior to PCI, followed by continuous infusion for 12 hours. [59] It attains a peak plasma concentration 2 hours after dosage with a half-life of 0.5 hours. [60] The primary mechanism of drug elimination is unknown but catabolism or proteolytic degradation with negligible renal excretion is expected. Current manufacturer recommendations state that dosing modifications are not necessary in patients with renal or hepatic impairment. [61]

Adverse Effects

Adverse effects of abciximab include bleeding (particularly if used in conjunction with other anticoagulant therapy) as well as blurred vision and orthostatic hypotension. Less common side effects include thrombocytopenia and rare side effects includes anaphylaxis, hypotension, chest pain, shortness of breath, bradycardia and arrhythmias. [58]

Reversal Agents

To date, there have been no antidotes identified for use in the event of an acute bleed in patients on abciximab. Current guidelines recommend platelet transfusions in adjunct to supportive management in the event of an acute bleed in patients on abciximab. [58]

Monitoring

Prior to infusion of abciximab, baseline values for aPTT, hemoglobin (Hgb), hematocrit (Hct) and platelet should be obtained. Platelet counts should be obtained 2-4 hours after bolus and at 24 hours or prior to discharge. [58]

Recommended Withholding Period Prior to Endoscopic Procedures

Abciximab should be discontinued 12-24 hours prior to any procedure, with 24 hours being preferred. [62]

EFTIFIBATIDE (INTEGRILIN®)

Eptifibatide is approved for its use in patients with acute coronary syndrome, including both those patients who are to be managed medically and those undergoing PCI (with or without stent placement). [63]

Pharmacokinetics and Pharmacodynamics

Eptifbatide is a cyclic heptapeptide that inhibits platelet aggregation by binding to the GPIIb/IIIa receptor. Eptifibatide is dosed as an intravenous bolus followed by continuous infusion and attains a peak plasma concentration within 4-6 hours after dosage. It has a half-life of 2.5 hours. The kidneys account for approximately 50% of drug clearance, therefore dosing should be adjusted for renal impairment as defined as a CrCl <50mL/min. Current manufacturer recommendations state that dosing modifications are not necessary in patients with hepatic impairment. [63]

Adverse Effects

Adverse effects of eptifibatide include bleeding (particularly if used in conjunction with other anticoagulant) as well as blurred vision, abdominal pain, confusion and orthostatic hypotension. Rare side effects include thrombocytopenia, anaphylaxis, hypotension, chest pain, shortness of breath, paralysis, tachycardia, palpitations, and arrhythmias. [63]

Reversal Agents

To date, there are no available reversal agents that can be used in the event of an acute bleed in patients on eptifibatide. Current guidelines recommend platelet transfusions in adjunct to supportive management. [63]

Monitoring

Prior to infusion of eftifibatide, baseline values for aPTT, hemoglobin (Hgb), hematocrit (Hct) and platelet should be obtained. There are no formal monitoring recommendations for eptifibatide after the baseline parameters, however if at any point the platelet count decreases below 100,000 then eptifibatide infusion should be discontinued. [63]

Recommended Withholding Period Prior to Endoscopic Procedures

Eptifibatide should be discontinued 2-4 hours prior to any procedure where therapeutic intervention is anticipated or planned. [62]

TIROFIBAN (AGGRASTAT®)

Tirofiban is a reversible glycoprotein IIb/IIIa antagonist that is approved for its use in patients with acute coronary syndrome, including both those patients who are to be managed medically and those individuals undergoing percutaneous coronary intervention (with or without stent placement). [64]

Pharmacokinetics and Pharmacodynamics

Tirofiban is a synthetic, non-peptide reversible inhibitor that binds to the GIIb/IIIa receptor inhibiting platelet aggregation. Tirofiban is dosed as an intravenous bolus that is to be continued through and following angiography. It reaches a peak plasma concentration 2 hours after dosage with a half-life of 2 hours. Renal pathways account for approximately 65% of the clearance. Renal dosing is therefore required in patients with a CrCl <30mL/min. Current manufacturer recommendations state that dosing modifications are not necessary in patients with hepatic impairment. [64]

Adverse Effects

Adverse effects of tirofiban include bleeding (particularly if used in conjunction with other anticoagulant therapy) as well as headache, abdominal pain, and orthostatic hypotension. Rare side effects include thrombocytopenia, anaphylaxis, chest pain, shortness of breath, and bradycardia. [64]

Reversal Agents

To date, there have been no antidotes identified for use in the event of an acute bleed in patients on tirofiban. Tirofibran has a relatively short half-life and its platelet effects dissipate rather quickly. When immediate reversal is required currently guidelines recommend platelet transfusions in adjunct to supportive management in the setting of an acute bleed. Tirofibran is dialyzable therefore when immediate reversal is required hemodialysis should also be considered. [64]

Monitoring

Prior to infusion of tirofiban, baseline values for aPTT, hemoglobin (Hgb), hematocrit (Hct) and platelet should be obtained. There are no formal monitoring recommendations for tirofiban after the baseline parameters, however if at any point the platelet count decreases below 90,000 (following repeat platelet counts to exclude pseudothrombocytopenia), tirofiban infusion should be discontinued. [64]

Recommended Withholding Period Prior to Endoscopic Procedures

Tirofiban can be stopped at the start of the procedure without harmful hematologic effects. [62]

HEPARIN

Pharmacokinetics and Pharmacodynamics

Heparin is a sulfated polysaccharide that binds to antithrombin III causing a conformational change and resulting in its activation. Now activated, antithrombin III inactivates thrombin and other proteases involved in the coagulation cascade, most notably factor Xa. The net result is the prevention of fibrin formation and the inhibition of thrombin-induced activation of platelets as well as factors V and VIII. [65] Figure 7 depicts the effect of heparin on the formation of a thrombus.

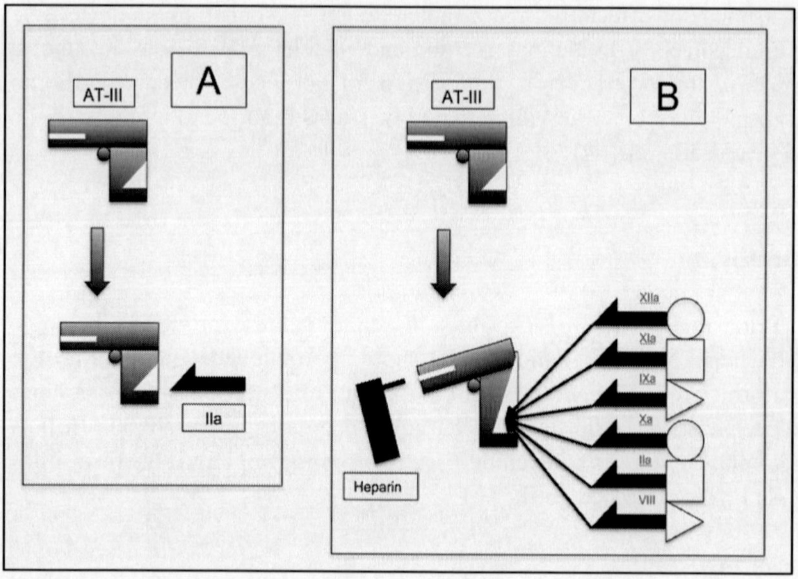

Figure 7. Mechanism of action of heparin. [91]

Heparin is indicated for treatment of atrial fibrillation with embolization, diagnosis and treatment of acute and chronic consumption coagulopathies, prevention of clotting in arterial and heart surgery, prophylaxis and treatment of peripheral arterial embolism, and prophylaxis and treatment of venous thromboembolism. Heparin attains a peak plasma concentration 2-4 hours after dosage with a half-life of 1.5 hours that is dose dependent. [66] It is dosed as an intravenous drip with or without a bolus dependent on the clinical scenario.

In addition, it can be dosed twice daily or thrice daily subcutaneously for DVT prophylaxis. Heparin is eliminated from the body via two mechanisms. The first is a dose dependent endothelial cell and macrophage mediated depolymerization, which accounts for the large molecular weight molecules, and the second is a dose independent elimination by the kidneys, which accounts for the low molecular weight molecules. [67]

Adverse Effects

Adverse effects of heparin include bleeding (particularly if used in conjunction with other anticoagulant therapy) as well as well as elevation in aminotransferases. Rare side effects include thrombocytopenia, hyperkalemia (through aldosterone suppression) and osteoporosis. [68] Heparin induced thrombocytopenia (both immune mediated and non-immune mediated subtypes) occur within 5-14 days after the initiation of heparin therapy. [69] Platelet counts typically begin to increase 2-3 days upon discontinuing heparin and usually to return to baseline levels within 4-10 days. In the immune-mediated subtype, the antibody disappears within 2-3 months after cessation of therapy. It is important to note that platelet transfusions should be avoided in cases of heparin-induced thrombocytopenia as it can further exacerbate the condition. [70]

Reversal Agents

In the event of an acute bleed in patients on heparin protamine sulfate is the standard of care with a dose of 1mg/100 units of heparin required in the previous 2-3 hours. When immediate reversal is required recombinant factor VIIa can be considered in addition to protamine sulfate. [71]

Monitoring

Prior to infusion of heparin, baseline values for aPTT, hemoglobin (Hgb), hematocrit (Hct) and platelet should be obtained. aPTT should be followed every 6-8 hours until 2 consecutive therapeutic PTT levels are achieved at a constant rate at which point aPTT should be checked daily. In addition, platelet counts should be monitored daily while on heparin and if any point the platelet count decreases below 100,000 or reduces by 50% over 24 hours (following repeat platelet counts to exclude pseudothrombocytopenia), heparin infusion should be discontinued and a heparin-induced thrombocytopenia work up should be initiated. [72]

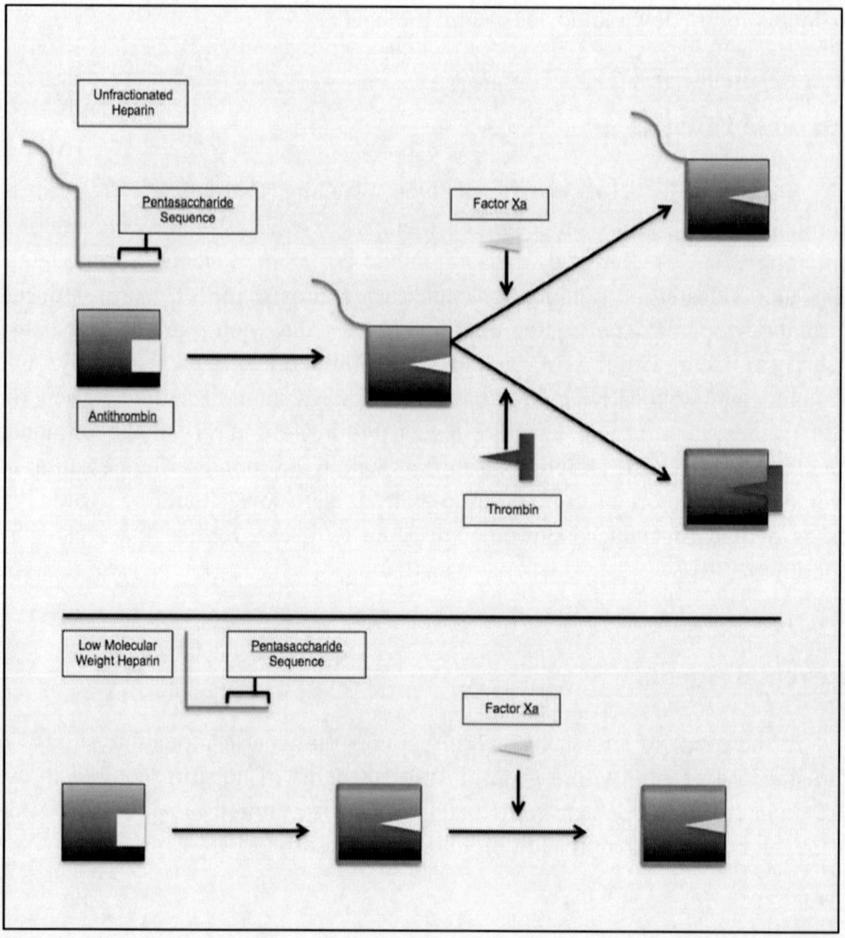

Figure 8. Difference in molecular size between heparin and low molecular weight heparin. [92]

Recommended Withholding Period Prior to Endoscopic Procedures

Current recommendations are that heparin should be discontinued 4-6 hours prior to any procedure. [73]

Low Molecular Weight Heparin

Low molecular weight heparins have a mechanism of action similar to that of heparin, the only difference being its molecular size. Figure 8 depicts the difference in molecular size between heparin and low molecular weight heparin.

Dalteparin (Fragmin®)

Dalteparin is a low molecular weight heparin approved for its use in prophylaxis of ischemic complications in the setting of unstable angina and non-Q-wave myocardial infarction, prophylaxis of deep vein thrombosis in abdominal surgery, hip replacement surgery or medical patients with severely restricted mobility during acute illness, and extended treatment of symptomatic venous thromboembolism to reduce recurrence in patients with cancer. [74]

Pharmacokinetics and Pharmacodynamics

Dalteparin is a low molecular weight heparin that binds to antithrombin III. In doing so, the resulting complex enhances the inhibition of thrombin and other proteases particularly factor Xa. Dalteparin attains a peak plasma concentration within 3-5 hours after dosage with a half-life of 2.2 hours and bioavailability of 87+/-6%. It is dosed as a once daily subcutaneous injection for prophylaxis and treatment of deep vein thrombosis or twice-daily subcutaneous injection for treatment of angina pectoris or myocardial infarction. The primary mechanism by which dalteparin is cleared from the plasma is via renal excretion therefore dose adjustments are required in patients with renal impairment (defined as a CrCl <30 mL/min). [74]

Adverse Effects

Adverse effects of dalteparin include bleeding (particularly if used in conjunction with other anticoagulant therapy) as well as asymptomatic elevation of aminotransferases and thrombocytopenia (common in patients with cancer). Rare side effects include thrombocytopenia (in the general patient population) and anaphylaxis. [74]

Reversal Agents

To date, there have been no antidotes identified for use in the event of an acute bleed in patients on dalteparin. In the event of an acute bleed in patients on dalteparin, protamine sulfate is the standard of care with a dose of 1mg / 100 units of dalteparin required in the previous 8 hours. When immediate reversal is required recombinant factor VIIa can be considered in addition to protamine sulfate. [71]

Monitoring

Prior to infusion of dalteparin, baseline values for aPTT, hemoglobin (Hgb), hematocrit (Hct) and platelet should be obtained. In addition, platelet counts should be monitored routinely while on dalteparin to monitor for thrombocytopenia. If at any point platelet counts decrease below 100,000 (following repeat platelet counts to exclude pseudothromboytyopenia), dalteparin should be discontinued and a thrombocytopenia work up should be initiated. Routine coagulation tests including aPTT and PT are relatively insensitive and therefore unsuitable for monitoring the anticoagulant effect. Anti-Factor Xa may be used to monitor the anticoagulant effect of dalteparin, and should be considered in patients with severe renal impairment, if any abnormal coagulation parameters or bleeding occurs while on dalteparin. [71]

Recommended Withholding Period Prior to Endoscopic Procedures

Current recommendations are that dalteparin should be discontinued 24 hours prior to any procedure. [75]

ENOXAPARIN (LOVENOX, XAPARIN, CLEXANE®)

Enoxaparin is a low molecular weight heparin approved for its use in prophylaxis of deep vein thrombosis in abdominal surgery, hip replacement surgery, knee replacement surgery or medical patients with severe restricted mobility during an acute illness, inpatient and outpatient treatment of an acute DVT without pulmonary embolism, inpatient treatment of an acute DVT with pulmonary embolism, and treatment of acute ST-segment elevation myocardial infarction (STEMI) managed medically or with subsequent percutaneous coronary intervention. [76]

Pharmacokinetics and Pharmacodynamics

Enoxaparin is a low molecular weight heparin that binds to antithrombin III. In doing so, the resulting complex enhances the inhibition of thrombin and other proteases particularly factor Xa. Dosed as a once daily or twice-daily subcutaneous injection, enoxaparin attains a peak plasma concentration within 3-5 hours after dosage with a half-life of 4.5 hours and bioavailability of 92%. The primary mechanism by which enoxaparin is cleared from the plasma is via renal excretion therefore dose adjustments are required in patients with renal impairment (defined as a CrCl <30 mL/min). [76]

Adverse Effects

Adverse effects of enoxaparin include bleeding (particularly if used in conjunction with other anticoagulant therapy) as well as asymptomatic elevation of aminotransferases, anemia, thrombocytopenia, nausea and vomiting. Rare side effects include thrombocytopenia. [76]

Reversal Agents

To date, there have been no antidotes identified for use in the event of an acute bleed in patients on enoxaparin. In the event of an acute bleed in patients on enoxaparin, protamine sulfate is the standard of care with a dose of 1mg/1mg of enoxaparin required in the previous 8 hours. When immediate reversal is required recombinant factor VIIa can be considered in addition to protamine sulfate. [71]

Monitoring

Prior to infusion of enoxaparin, baseline values for aPTT, hemoglobin (Hgb), hematocrit (Hct) and platelet should be obtained. In addition, platelet counts should be monitored routinely while on enoxaparin to monitor for thrombocytopenia. If at any point platelet counts decrease below 100,000 (following repeat platelet counts to exclude pseudothromboytyopenia), enoxparin should be discontinued and a thrombocytopenia work up should be initiated. Routine coagulation tests including aPTT and PT are relatively insensitive and therefore unsuitable for monitoring the anticoagulant effect. Anti-Factor Xa, also referred to as the "low molecular weight heparin assay" may be used to monitor the anticoagulant effect of enoxaparin, and should be considered in patients with severe renal impairment, patients who are at the extremes of weight (<45kg or >150 kg) or if any abnormal coagulation parameters or bleeding occurs while on enoxaparin. The draw time of the assay is generally 4 hours post-dose of enoxaparin as this measures its peak activity. [76]

Recommended Withholding Period Prior to Endoscopic Procedures

Current recommendations are that enoxaparin should be discontinued at least 24 hours prior to any procedure. [75]

FONDAPARINUX (ARIXTRA®)

Fondaparinux is a low molecular weight heparin approved for its use in prophylaxis of deep vein thrombosis in abdominal surgery, hip replacement surgery, knee replacement surgery or medical patients with severe restricted mobility during an acute illness, or treatment of DVT or acute pulmonary embolism when administered in conjunction with warfarin. [77]

Pharmacokinetics and Pharmacodynamics

Fondaparinux is a low molecular weight heparin that binds to antithrombin III. In doing so, the resulting complex enhances the inhibition of thrombin and other proteases particularly factor Xa. Dosed as a once daily subcutaneous injection, fondaparinux attains a peak plasma concentration within 3 hours after dosage with a half-life of 17-21 hours and bioavailability of 100%. The primary mechanism by which fondaparinux is cleared from the plasma is via renal excretion therefore dose adjustments are required in patients with renal impairment (defined as a CrCl <30 mL/min). [77]

Adverse Effects

Adverse effects of fondapariunux include bleeding (particularly if used in conjunction with other anticoagulants) as well as asymptomatic elevation of aminotransferases, anemia, thrombocytopenia, nausea and vomiting. [77]

Reversal Agents

To date, there have been no antidotes identified for use in the setting of an acute bleed in patients on fondaparinux. In the event of an acute bleed in patients on fondaparinux, protamine sulfate is the standard of care. When immediate reversal is required recombinant factor VIIa can be considered in addition to protamine sulfate. [71]

Monitoring

Prior to infusion of fondaparinux, baseline values for aPTT, hemoglobin (Hgb), hematocrit (Hct) and platelet should be obtained. In addition, platelet counts should be monitored routinely while on fondaparinux to monitor for thrombocytopenia. If at any point platelet counts decrease below 100,000 (following repeat platelet counts to exclude pseudothromboytyopenia), fondaparinux should be discontinued and a thrombocytopenia work up should be initiated. Routine coagulation tests including aPTT and PT are relatively insensitive and therefore unsuitable for monitoring the anticoagulant effect. Anti-Factor Xa may be used to monitor the anticoagulant effect of fondaparinux, and should be considered in patients with severe renal impairment, if any abnormal coagulation parameters or bleeding occurs while on fondaparinux. [77]

Recommended Withholding Period Prior to Endoscopic Procedures

Current recommendations are that fondaparinux should be discontinued at least 24 hours prior to any procedure. [75]

Discussion

The development and introduction of new anticoagulant and antiplatelet therapies has been explosive. As patients who use the medications have gastrointestinal disease or need emergent or elective endoscopic procedures, it is critical for patient safety that gastroenterologists fully understand the pharmacology so as to best manage the clinical impact of usage from a gastrointestinal perspective. The pharmacokinetics, dosing, reversal agents and recommendations on pre-procedural withholding periods for warfarin and the more modern agents are summarized as best practice recommendations in Table 6.

Table 6. Best practice recommendations

Class	Agent	Peak (Hours)	Half-Life (Hours)	Bioavailability (%)	Dosing	Reversal Agents (See below for HASHTI[42])	Recommendations to Discontinue Prior to Procedure
Vitamin K Antagonist	Warfarin	72-96	20-60	100	Daily	1. Vitamin K (IV/PO) 1-10mg *Takes 6 (IV) to 24 (PO) hours to reverse 2. Fresh Frozen Plasma 10-30mL/kg (1 unit = ~250 mL) 3. Prothombin Complex Concentrates 25-50 units/kg IV	Discontinue 5 days prior to procedure
Xa Inhibitor	Rivaroxaban (Xarelto®)	2.5-4	5-9 (9-13 if elderly)	80	Daily or BID	1. Supportive Treatment 2. Factor VIIa 3. Prothombin Complex Concentrates 25-50 units/kg IV	Discontinue 24 hours prior to procedure
	Apixaban (Eliquis®)	3	8-13	~66	BID	1. Supportive Treatment 2. Factor VIIa 3. Prothombin Complex Concentrates 25-50 units/kg IV	Discontinue 24 hours prior to procedure if low risk of bleeding or 48 hours prior to procedure if high risk bleeding
Direct Thrombin Inhibitor	Dabigatran (Pradaxa®)	2-3	13-27 (Depending on CrCl – refer to Table 1)	6.5	Daily or BID	1. Supportive Blood Products / HASHTI[42] 2. Prothombin Complex Concentrates 3. Consider rVIIa 4. Hemodialysis	Refer to Table 7
	Bivalirudin (Angiomax®)	0.5-3	0.5	100	Intravenous	1. Supportive Blood Products / HASHTI[42] 2. Consider rVIIa (90mcg/kg for up to 2 doses) 3. Hemodialysis	Discontinue prior to induction of anesthesia in a patient with normal renal function
	Argatroban	1-3	39 - 51 (minutes)	100	Intravenous	1. Supportive Blood Products / HASHTI[42] 2. Prothombin Complex Concentrates 3. Consider rVIIa 4. Hemodialysis	Discontinue 4-6 hours prior to induction of anesthesia in a patient with normal hepatic function

Table 6. (Continued)

Thienopyridine Antiplatelet Agent	Clopidogrel (Plavix®)	1	7-8	>50	Daily	1. HASHTI[42] 2. Platelet Transfusion 3.Case Reports of Methylprednisolone and DDAVP	Discontinue 5-10 days prior to procedure
	Ticlopidine (Ticlid®)	2	12	>80	BID	1. HASHTI[42] 2. Platelet Transfusion	Discontinue 5-10 days prior to procedure
	Prasugrel (Effient®)	0.5	2-15	>79	Daily	1. HASHTI[42] 2. Platelet Transfusion	Discontinue 5-10 days prior to procedure
	Ticagrelor (Brillinta®)	1.5	7-8.5	>36	Daily or BID	1. HASHTI[42] 2. Platelet Transfusion	Discontinue 5-10 days prior to procedure
	Dipyrimadole (Persantine®)	1.25	7-10	50-75	QID	1. HASHTI[42] 2. Platelet Transfusion 3. Aminophylline for Dipyrimadole overdose	Discontinue 7 days prior to procedure
	(Aggrenox® [Extrended Release Dipyrimadole + Aspirin])	2	13.6	50-75	BID	1. HASHTI[42] 2. Platelet Transfusion	Discontinue 7 days prior to procedure
Glycoprotein IIB/IIIA Inhibitors	Abciximab (ReoPro®)	2	0.5	100	Intravenous	1. HASHTI[42] 2. Platelet Transfusion	12 – 24 hours prior to procedure (24 ideal)
	Eptifibatide (Integrilin®)	4-6	2.5	100	Intravenous	1. HASHTI[42] 2. Platelet Transfusion	2 – 4 hours prior to procedure
	Tirofiban (Aggrastat®)	2	2	100	Intravenous	1. HASHTI[42] 2. Platelet Transfusion 3. Dialysis	Can be stopped at the moment of skin incision without harmful effects.
Low Molecular Weight Heparin	Dalteparin (Fragmin®)	3-5	2.2	87	Subcutaneous	1. HASHTI[42] 2. Protamine sulfate (1mg/100 units Dalteparin in previous 8 hours)	Last dose should be given 24 hours prior to procedure

Evaluation of Long Term Anticoagulant Therapy) trial, which randomized over 18,000 patients, demonstrated that a 150-mg dose of dabigatran was superior to warfarin for overall stroke and systemic embolism prevention. [79] Table 7 below depicts the notable outcomes from the RE-LY trial and particular attention should be given to bleeding risk. Further evaluation of bleeding risk shows dabigatran to be safer when compared to warfarin in terms of total bleeds, major bleeds and life-threatening bleeds however dabigatran is associated with a higher risk of major GI bleeds as illustrated in Figure 9. The RE-LY trial was a landmark trial that led to the approval of dabigatran in patients with non-valvular atrial fibrillation and heralded the entry of other anticoagulants.

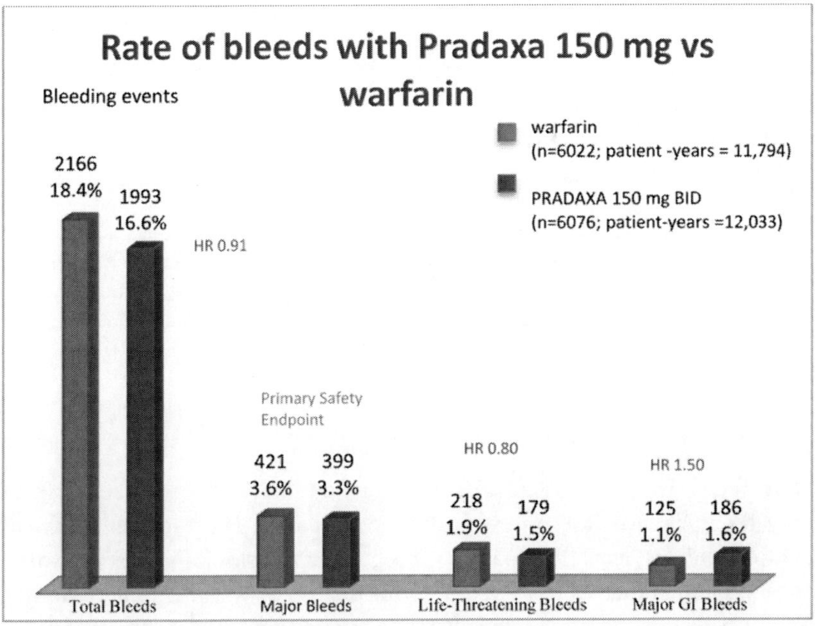

Figure 9. Adverse outcomes from RE-LY trial. [94]

Similarly, the ROCKET AF (Rivaroxaban Once Daily Oral Direct Factor Xa Inhibition Compared with Vitamin K Antagonism for Prevention of Stroke and Embolism Trial in Atrial Fibrillation) trial, which randomized 14,264 patients with a primary endpoint of stroke or embolism prevention in patients with atrial fibrillation, demonstrated rivaroxaban was non-inferior to warfarin. Further evaluation of bleeding outcomes from this study trial showed that major GI bleeds were more common in the rivaroxaban group, with 224 events (3.2%), as compared to the 154 events in the warfarin group (2.2%, P<0.001) [80] (see Table 8).

Table 8. Adverse outcomes from ROCKET-AF Trial [80]

Major bleeding by site[1]	Rivaroxaban (n=7,111)	Warfarin (n=7,125)
Major bleeding, no. (%)	395 (5.55)	386 (5.42)
Gastrointestinal (upper, lower and rectal)[2]	224 (3.15)	154 (2.16)
Intracranial[3]	55 (0.77)	84 (1.18)
Intraparenchymal[3]	37 (0.52)	56 (0.79)
Non-traumatic[3]	33 (0.46)	54 (1.76)
Traumatic	4 (0.06)	2 (0.03)
Intraventricular	2 (0.03)	4 (0.06)
Subdural hematoma	0	1 (0.01)
Subarachnoid	4 (0.06)	1 (0.01)
Epidural hematoma	0	1 (0.01)
Macrscopic hematuria	26 (0.37)	21 (0.29)
Bleeding associated with non-cardiac surgery	19 (0.27)	26 (0.36)
Intraocular/Retinal	17 (0.24)	24 (0.34)
Intra-articular	16 (0.23)	21 (0.29)
Epistaxis	13 (0.18)	14 (0.20)

Key
[1]Site based on blinded adjudication
[2]Combined gastrointestinal bleed rate P<0.001
[3]P<0.05

The recent trial data has [79,80] clarified the best practice targeted strategy for the use of these new oral anticoagulants. These newer regimens appeal to clinicians, as well as patients, because of the ease of use as they offer less oversight than that which is required for the use of warfarin. Endoscopists, however, need to be cognizant that these new agents seem to higher predilection of GI bleeding. [79,80] Unfortunately to date there is only anecdotal evidence supporting the use of any reversal agents in the setting of an acute GI bleed for these newer anticoagulants or antiplatelet agents. Although reversal agents may be in the pipeline, these agents are not available, the pragmatic issue is that gastroenterologists continue to witness major GI bleeding on these newer anticoagulants and therefore best practice strategies for management are needed not only for prevention for elective procedures, but also for management of acute events.

Clearly it is well recognized that the temporary discontinuance of these agents is safe for elective procedures when at least 6 months after stent placement, but at least for diagnostic procedures the cardiovascular complications of stopping these agents may outweigh the bleeding risks. It is therefore, strongly recommended that the gastroenterologist/endoscopist never be the one to instruct the patient to stop any anticoagulant or antiplatelet therapy. This should be a recommendation pending the patient finalizing approval by the prescriber of these agents- typically the cardiologist, neurologist, and vascular surgeon or primary care provider. Additionally, the necessity for approved reversal agents for these new drugs remains of utmost concern, particularly in dealing with emergent bleeding complications. The recommendations presented in this review are based on the best evidence available at this time. Clearly new guidelines for best practice recommendations from both the cardiology and gastrointestinal national societies addressing management for elective and emergent endoscopic procedures as well as management for acute gastrointestinal bleeding in patients on these agents are needed.

Summary Points

1. The pharmacologic agents used for anticoagulation continues to expand, as do the clinical indications for its usage.
2. Currently, there is limited data on drug-interactions with other agents or herbal supplements with regards to the new oral anticoagulants.
3. Lack of reversal agents is also of significant concern. The protocols discussed are the most up to date, however when dealing with such agents close attention should be paid to any developments in reversal agents or updated protocols.
4. The pharmacodynamics and pharmacokinetics as well as reveral and withholding protococols for each agent are summarized in Table 6.

References

[1] Holster IL, Valkhoff VE, Kuipers EJ, Tjwa ET. New oral anticoagulants increase risk for gastrointestinal bleeding: a systematic review and meta-analysis. *Gastroenterology*. 2013;145(1):105-112.e15.

[2] Clemetson KJ. Platelets and primary haemostasis. Thromb Res. 2012;129(3):220-4.

[3] Pallister C, Watson M. *Haematology.* Scion; 2011.

[4] Whitlon DS, Sadowski JA, Suttie JW. Mechanism of coumarin action: significance of vitamin K epoxide reductase inhibition. *Biochemistry.* 1978;17(8):1371-7.

[5] Available at: http://www.coumadin.com/html/index.htm. Accessed July 11, 2013.

[6] Available at: http://www.medscape.com/viewarticle/406896_2. Accessed July 11, 2013.

[7] Kuruvilla M, Gurk-turner C. A review of warfarin dosing and monitoring. Proc (Bayl Univ Med Cent). 2001;14(3):305-6.

[8] Available at: http://emedicine.medscape.com/article/285265-overview. Accessed July 11, 2013.

[9] Wilkens M, Krishnaswamy S. The contribution of factor Xa to exosite-dependent substrate recognition by prothrombinase. *J Biol Chem.* 2002;277(11):9366-74.

[10] Nesheim ME, Taswell JB, Mann KG. The contribution of bovine Factor V and Factor Va to the activity of prothrombinase. *J Biol Chem.* 1979;254(21):10952-62.

[11] Available at: http://www.xareltohcp.com/sites/default/files/pdf/medication_guide#zoom=100. Accessed June 2, 2013.

[12] Bauer KA. Reversal of antithrombotic agents. *Am J Hematol.* 2012;87 Suppl 1:S119-26.

[13] Kaatz S, Kouides PA, Garcia DA, et al. Guidance on the emergent reversal of oral thrombin and factor Xa inhibitors. *Am J Hematol.* 2012;87 Suppl 1:S141-5.

[14] Marlu R, Hodaj E, Pernod G. Letter by Marlu et al regarding article, "reversal of rivaroxaban and dabigatran by prothrombin complex concentrate: a randomized, placebo-controlled, crossover study in healthy subjects". *Circulation.* 2012;125(16):e615.

[15] Available at: http://www.xareltohcp.com/sites/default/files/pdf/xarelto_0#zoom=100. Accessed April 30, 2013

[16] Kubitza D, Becka M, Mueck W, et al. Effects of renal impairment on the pharmacokinetics, pharmacodynamics and safety of rivaroxaban, an oral, direct Factor Xa inhibitor. *Br J Clin Pharmacol.* 2010;70(5):703-12.

[17] Available at: http://www.medscape.com/viewarticle/776846. Accessed July 11, 2013.

[18] Agnelli G, Buller HR, Cohen A, et al. Apixaban for extended treatment of venous thromboembolism. *N Engl J Med.* 2013;368(8):699-708.

[19] Available at: http://packageinserts.bms.com/pi/pi_eliquis. Accessed July 11, 2013

[20] Available at: http://reference.medscape.com/drug/eliquis-apixaban-999805. Accessed July 11, 2013.

[21] Warkentin TE. Bivalent direct thrombin inhibitors: hirudin and bivalirudin. *Best Pract Res Clin Haematol.* 2004;17(1):105-25.

[22] Rosenfeld SA, Nadeau D, Tirado J, Hollis GF, Knabb RM, Jia S. Production and purification of recombinant hirudin expressed in the methylotrophic yeast Pichia pastoris. *Protein Expr Purif.* 1996;8(4):476-82.

[23] Januzzi JL, Jang IK. Heparin induced thrombocytopenia: diagnosis and contemporary antithrombin management. *J Thromb Thrombolysis.* 1999;7(3):259-64.

[24] Greinacher A. Lepirudin: a bivalent direct thrombin inhibitor for anticoagulation therapy. *Expert Rev Cardiovasc Ther.* 2004;2(3):339-57.

[25] Dornan RI. Hirudin and its reversal. *Br J Anaesth.* 2002;89(3):524.

[26] Koster A, Merkle F, Hansen R, et al. Elimination of recombinant hirudin by modified ultrafiltration during simulated cardiopulmonary bypass: assessment of different filter systems. *Anesth Analg.* 2000;91(2):265-9.

[27] Petros S. Lepirudin in the management of patients with heparin-induced thrombocytopenia. Biologics. 2008;2(3):481-90.

[28] Available at: http://www.angiomax.com/downloads/Angiomax%20US%20PI-%20PN%201601-15.pdf. Accessed July 11, 2013.

[29] Harrington RA, Becker RC, Cannon CP, et al. Antithrombotic therapy for non-ST-segment elevation acute coronary syndromes: American College of Chest Physicians Evidence-Based Clinical Practice Guidelines (8th Edition). *Chest.* 2008;133(6 Suppl):670S-707S.

[30] Stone GW, Witzenbichler B, Guagliumi G, et al. Bivalirudin during primary PCI in acute myocardial infarction. *N Engl J Med.* 2008;358(21):2218-30.

[31] Haines ST, Bussey HI. Thrombosis and the pharmacology of antithrombotic agents. *Ann Pharmacother.* 1995;29(9):892-905.

[32] Available at: http://www.itxm.org/tmu/tmu2007/2007ISSUE6. Accessed February 22, 2013.

[33] Young G, Yonekawa KE, Nakagawa PA, Blain RC, Lovejoy AE, Nugent DJ. Recombinant activated factor VII effectively reverses the anticoagulant effects of heparin, enoxaparin, fondaparinux, argatroban, and bivalirudin ex vivo as measured using thromboelastography. *Blood Coagul Fibrinolysis.* 2007;18(6):547-53.

[34] Newman MF, Fleisher LA, Fink MM. Perioperative Medicine, Managing for Outcome. Saunders; 2008. Chapter 27: Perioperative Management of Bleeding and Transfusion.

[35] Available at: http://bidocs.boehringer-ingelheim.com/BIWebAccess/ViewServlet.ser?docBase=renetnt&folderPath=/Prescribing Information/PIs/Pradaxa/Patient Info/PradaxaMedGuide. Accessed April 30, 2013.

[36] Schulman S, Kearon C, Kakkar AK, et al. Extended use of dabigatran, warfarin, or placebo in venous thromboembolism. *N Engl J Med.* 2013; 368(8):709-18.

[37] Hankey GJ, Eikelboom JW. Dabigatran etexilate: a new oral thrombin inhibitor. Circulation. 2011;123(13):1436-50.

[38] Available at: http://www.pradaxapro.com/adverse-reactions.jsp. Accessed September 8, 2013.

[39] Available at: http://healthcare.utah.edu/thrombosis/newagents/TS.Dabi_Bleeding. Accessed April 30, 2013.

[40] Chang DN, Dager WE, Chin AI. Removal of dabigatran by hemodialysis. Am J Kidney Dis. 2013;61(3):487-9.

[41] Woulfe D, Yang J, Brass L. ADP and platelets: the end of the beginning. *J Clin Invest.* 2001;107(12):1503-5.

[42] Available at: http://reference.medscape.com/drug/ticlid-ticlopidine-342184. Accessed July 11, 2013.

[43] Savi P, Herbert JM. Clopidogrel and ticlopidine: P2Y12 adenosine diphosphate-receptor antagonists for the prevention of atherothrombosis. *Semin Thromb Hemost.* 2005;31(2):174-83.

[44] Available at: http://www.hematology.org/practice/guidelines/7243.aspx &ei=q9neUaSEGOatigKs9oDQCw&usg=AFQjCNFc9umeh1fPpTKWd

dZo7dhq9NCRWQ&sig2=Qa57N4Iab8Xn29pQkpiPHA. Accessed July 11, 2013.

[45] Available at: http://packageinserts.bms.com/pi/pi_plavix.pdf. Accessed February 24, 2013.

[46] Douglas IJ, Evans SJ, Hingorani AD, et al. Clopidogrel and interaction with proton pump inhibitors: comparison between cohort and within person study designs. *BMJ.* 2012;345(jul10 1):e4388.

[47] Stein PD, Schünemann HJ, Dalen JE, Gutterman D. Antithrombotic therapy in patients with saphenous vein and internal mammary artery bypass grafts: the Seventh ACCP Conference on Antithrombotic and Thrombolytic Therapy. *Chest.* 2004;126(3 Suppl):600S-608S

[48] Available at: http://pi.lilly.com/us/effient.pdf. Accessed July 11, 2013

[49] Wiviott SD, Braunwald E, Mccabe CH, et al. Prasugrel versus clopidogrel in patients with acute coronary syndromes. *N Engl J Med.* 2007;357(20):2001-15.

[50] O'connor S, Montalescot G, Collet JP. The P2Y(12) receptor as a target of antithrombotic drugs. *Purinergic Signal.* 2011;7(3):325-32.

[51] Varenhorst C, James S, Erlinge D, et al. Genetic variation of CYP2C19 affects both pharmacokinetic and pharmacodynamic responses to clopidogrel but not prasugrel in aspirin-treated patients with coronary artery disease. *Eur Heart J.* 2009;30(14):1744-52.

[52] Available at: http://www.effienthcp.com/Pages/clinical-guidelines.aspx. Accessed July 11, 2013.

[53] Available at: http://www.astrazeneca-us.com/cgi-bin/az_pi.cgi?product=brilinta&country=us&popup=no. Accessed July 11, 2013.

[54] Wallentin L, Becker RC, Budaj A, et al. Ticagrelor versus clopidogrel in patients with acute coronary syndromes. *N Engl J Med.* 2009;361(11):1045-57.

[55] Capodanno D, Dharmashankar K, Angiolillo DJ. Mechanism of action and clinical development of ticagrelor, a novel platelet ADP P2Y12 receptor antagonist. *Expert Rev Cardiovasc Ther.* 2010;8(2):151-8.

[56] Available at: http://www.brilinta.com/questions-and-answers.aspx. Accessed February 24, 2013.

[57] Bennett JS. Structure and function of the platelet integrin alphaIIbbeta3. *J Clin Invest.* 2005;115(12):3363-9.

[58] Available at: http://www.reopro.com/Pages/index.aspx. Accessed February 24, 2013.

[59] Tcheng JE, Kandzari DE, Grines CL, et al. Benefits and risks of abciximab use in primary angioplasty for acute myocardial infarction: the Controlled Abciximab and Device Investigation to Lower Late Angioplasty Complications (CADILLAC) trial. *Circulation.* 2003;108(11):1316-23.

[60] Valgimigli M, Campo G, Tebaldi M, et al. Abciximab: a reappraisal of its use in coronary care. *Biologics.* 2008;2(1):29-39.

[61] Mager DE, Mascelli MA, Kleiman NS, Fitzgerald DJ, Abernethy DR. Simultaneous modeling of abciximab plasma concentrations and ex vivo pharmacodynamics in patients undergoing coronary angioplasty. *J Pharmacol Exp Ther.* 2003;307(3):969-76.

[62] Available at: http://mmcts.oxfordjournals.org/content/2010/1103/mmcts.2010.004580.full. Accessed July 12, 2013.

[63] Available at: http://www.integrilin.com/integrilin/index.html. Accessed July 12, 2013.

[64] Available at: http://www.medicure.com/aggrastat/aggrastat.html. Accessed July 12, 2013.

[65] Hirsh J, Anand SS, Halperin JL, Fuster V. Mechanism of action and pharmacology of unfractionated heparin. *Arterioscler Thromb Vasc Biol.* 2001;21(7):1094-6.

[66] Hirsh J, Anand SS, Halperin JL, Fuster V. AHA Scientific Statement: Guide to anticoagulant therapy: heparin: a statement for healthcare professionals from the American Heart Association. Arterioscler *Thromb Vasc Biol.* 2001;21(7):E9-9.

[67] Lehman CM, Frank EL. Laboratory Monitoring of Heparin Therapy: Partial Thromboplastin Time or Anti-Xa Assay?. Laboratory Medicine. 2009;40(1):47-51

[68] Available at: http://www.uptodate.com/contents/therapeutic-use-of-heparin-and-low-molecular-weight-heparin?source=search_result&search=heparin side effects& selected Title=1~150#H21. Accessed July 12, 2013.

[69] Baroletti SA, Goldhaber SZ. Heparin-induced thrombocytopenia. *Circulation.* 2006;114(8):e355-6.

[70] Franchini M. Heparin-induced thrombocytopenia: an update. *Thromb J.* 2005;3(1):14

[71] Warkentin TE, Crowther MA. Reversing anticoagulants both old and new. *Can J Anaesth.* 2002;49(6):S11-25.

[72] Available at: http://www.medscape.com/viewarticle/559442. Accessed July 12, 2013.

[73] Douketis JD, Spyropoulos AC, Spencer FA, et al. Perioperative management of antithrombotic therapy: Antithrombotic Therapy and Prevention of Thrombosis, 9th ed: American College of Chest Physicians Evidence-Based Clinical Practice Guidelines. *Chest.* 2012;141(2 Suppl):e326S-50S.

[74] Available at: http://www.fragmin.com. Accessed July 12, 2013.

[75] Jaffer AK. Perioperative management of warfarin and antiplatelet therapy. Cleve Clin J Med. 2009;76 Suppl 4(Suppl_4):S37-44.

[76] Available at: http://wwww.products.sanofi.us/lovenox/lovenox.html. Accessed July 12, 2013.

[77] Available at: http://www.gsksource.com/gskprm/en/US/adirect/gskprm?cmd=ProductDetailPage&product_id=1244136744215&featureKey=600552. Accessed July 12, 2013.

[78] Abraham NS. Novel oral anticoagulants and gastrointestinal bleeding: a case for cardiogastroenterology. *Clin Gastroenterol Hepatol.* 2013;11(4):324-8.

[79] Connolly SJ, Ezekowitz MD, Yusuf S, et al. Dabigatran versus warfarin in patients with atrial fibrillation. *N Engl J Med.* 2009;361(12):1139-51

[80] MR, Mahaffey KW, Garg J, et al. Rivaroxaban versus warfarin in nonvalvular atrial fibrillation. *N Engl J Med.* 2011;365(10):883-91.

[81] Available at: http://www.sharinginhealth.ca/biology/hemostasis.html. Accessed July 12, 2013.

[82] Available at: http://unont.com.ar/images/warfarin-mechanism-of-action-diagram-i19.gif. Accessed July 10, 2013

[83] Available at: http:// www.druginformation.com/RxDrugs/W/_di.warfarin%201.png. Accessed July 10, 2013

[84] Available at: http://www.emergency-medicine-tutorials.org/_/rsrc/1311294850923/Home/medical-3/haematology/anticoagulants-and-reversal/anticoagulant-agents/Warfarin%20Reversal%20Guidelines.jpg

[85] Accessed July 10, 2013

[86] Available at: http://www.zunis.org/anticoagulation_guidelines.htm. Accessed July 10, 2013

[87] Verma AK, Brighton TA. The direct factor Xa inhibitor rivaroxaban. *Med J Aust.* 2009;190(7):379-83.

[88] Linardi RL, Natalini CC. Multi-drug resistance (MDR1) gene and P-glycoprotein influence on pharmacokinetic and pharmacodymanic of therapeutic drugs. *Ciencia Rural* 36.1 (2006): 336-341.
[89] Baetz BE, Spinler SA. Dabigatran etexilate: an oral direct thrombin inhibitor for prophylaxis and treatment of thromboembolic diseases. *Pharmacotherapy.* 2008;28(11):1354-73
[90] Agrawal K, Bhatt DL. Antiplatelet therapy: Does prasugrel or ticagrelor suffice in patients with STEMI?. *Nat Rev Cardiol.* 2013;10(3):121-2.
[91] Gibler WB, Wilcox RG, Bode C, et al. Prospective use of platelet glycoprotein IIb/IIIa receptor blockers in the emergency department setting. *Eur J Emerg Med.* 1998;5(4):391-402.
[92] Available at: http://journals.prous.com/journals/dof/20022705/html/df270446/images/deligoparin_f2.gif. Accessed July 12, 2013.
[93] Whang PG, Lieberman JR. Low-molecular-weight herapin. *J Am Acad Orthop Surg.* 2002;10(5):299-302.
[94] Mcarthur MC, Dzintars EK, Phillips RB, Bushardt RL. Oral anticoagulation: a review of the current and emerging therapies. *JAAPA.* 2011;24(11):60-6.
[95] Available at: http://www.pradaxapro.com/safety.jsp. Accessed July 12, 2013

In: Clopidogrel
Editors: J. P. Alesci and A. Victorino
ISBN: 978-1-62948-336-8
© 2014 Nova Science Publishers, Inc.

Chapter 2

CLOPIDOGREL IN NEUROINTERVENTIONAL SURGERY: INDICATIONS, COMPLICATIONS, CHALLENGES AND METHODS FOR MONITORING RESPONSE

S. Hassan Akbari[1], Matthew R. Reynolds[1*] and Christopher J. Moran[1,2]

[1]Department of Neurological Surgery, Washington University School of Medicine, St. Louis, MO, US

[2]Department of Radiology, Mallinkrodt Institute of Radiology, Washington University School of Medicine, St. Louis, MO, US

ABSTRACT

Neurointerventional surgery has become an essential tool for the treatment of complex spinal and cerebrovascular diseases including cerebral aneurysms, dural arteriovenous fistulas (dAVF), arteriovenous malformations (AVM), carotid-cavernous fistulas, intra/extracranial atherosclerosis, intracranial thromboembolism, and neurological tumors. Techniques utilizing stents, coils, neuroembolic agents, flow-diverting devices, and combinations thereof are often used to treat these diverse

* Corresponding author: Matthew R. Reynolds, M.D., Ph.D., Barnes-Jewish Hospital, Department of Neurological Surgery, Campus Box 8057, 660 South Euclid Avenue, St. Louis, Missouri 63110; Email: ReynoldsM@wudosis.wustl.edu.

pathologies. While significant advances have been made in the field of neurointerventional surgery in recent years, the risk of peri-procedural thromboembolic complications (e.g., transient ischemic attack [TIA] and ischemic stroke) has been estimated at 8% due to the thrombogenic nature of the foreign guidewires and endovascular implants. Interventional cardiology—a field that utilizes similar endovascular techniques for stenting of diseased coronary vessels in myocardial ischemia/infarction—has demonstrated that post-procedural dual anti-platelet therapy (DAPT) with aspirin and clopidogrel minimizes the risk of thromboembolic complications and is more beneficial than aspirin therapy alone. Due to these findings, DAPT with aspirin (325 mg PO daily) and clopidogrel (75 mg PO daily), with or without a loading dose, has been recommended for neurointerventional procedures as well. However, limited research on the use of aspirin and clopidogrel for neurointerventional surgery currently exists in the literature to support these recommendations, and there are no formal guidelines for the use of anti-platelet agents in this setting. Additionally, recent data suggest that a large number of patients exhibit clopidogrel resistance, which may increase the rate of thromboembolic complications during endovascular procedures. As a result, novel anti-platelet agents are being increasingly utilized in this challenging patient population. The goal of this chapter is to highlight the use of clopidogrel in neurointerventional surgery, including indications for treatment, complications of treatment, challenges to the current treatment paradigm, methods for detection, and possible anti-platelet alternatives.

Keywords: Clopidogrel, Plavix, dual antiplatelet therapy, neurointerventional surgery, indications, complications, challenges, detection

ABBREVIATIONS

ADP	Adenosine Diphosphate
AVM	Arteriovenous Malformation
DAPT	Dual Antiplatelet Therapy
dAVF	Dural Arteriovenous Fistula
GI	Gastrointestinal
ICH	Intracerebral Hemorrhage
PED	Pipeline Embolization Device
PCI	Percutaneous Coronary Intervention
PFA	Platelet Function Assay
PPI	Proton Pump Inhibitor

STEMI	ST-Segment Elevation Myocardial Infarction
TIA	Transient Ischemic Attack
tPA	Tissue Plasminogen Activator

INTRODUCTION

Endovascular neurosurgery is a rapidly growing field that allows for minimally invasive therapeutic approaches to common neurosurgical pathologies. The endovascular technique utilizes remote access, commonly via the femoral vessels, for microcatheter advancement into the cerebral vasculature. Once the cerebral vessels have been accessed, various therapeutic tools may be utilized depending on the specific pathology to be addressed. These tools include coils, stents, embolic materials, balloons, flow-diverters, and medications.[1] Coils are often deployed into aneurysms where they serve as a nidus for thrombogenesis, thus occluding the aneurysm and removing it from the cerebral circulation. This treatment has been shown to substantially reduce the risk of re-rupture for previously ruptured aneurysms, and can also be used to treat non-ruptured aneurysms as well. Stents have been utilized not only in intracerebral atherosclerotic disease but also to assist in coiling procedures and the remodeling of broad necked aneurysms.[1] Recently, the Pipeline Embolic Device (PED; Ev3 Inc., Plymouth, Minnesota, USA) was developed as a tool to divert flow from the aneurysmal sac, thereby decreasing shear stress on the aneurysmal wall.[2] The PED achieves the goal of removing aneurysms from the cerebral circulation by remodeling the wall of the parent artery. Newer embolic materials including Onyx (Ev3 Inc., Plymouth, Minnesota, USA) can be useful in the treatment of AVMs, or can be used in combination with coils for neurointerventional procedures.[1, 3-5] Onyx—in addition to other embolic agents—has the ability to solidify inside AVMs and their major feeding arteries, thereby reducing flow to the diseased vessels and, subsequently, their risk of hemorrhage. Endovascular neurosurgery also allows for microcatheter-based delivery of various medications including intra-arterial tissue plasminogen activator (tPA) for ischemic stroke and calcium channel blockers for the treatment of cerebral vasospasm.[1, 6-7] These medications have significantly altered outcomes for patients with ischemic stroke and subarachnoid hemorrhage, respectively. Perhaps most importantly, neurointerventional surgery allows for the efficacious treatment of complex intracranial diseases with less morbidity and mortality than standard open microsurgical procedures. For example, in a recent, large prospective trial examining the functional outcomes of patients with an acutely ruptured intracerebral aneurysm treated by either microsurgical clipping or endovascular coiling, the authors found that endovascular coiling resulted in significantly fewer poor outcomes after one year (33.7% versus 23.2%, respectively; $p = 0.02$).[8]

INDICATIONS FOR CLOPIDOGREL IN NEUROINTERVENTIONAL SURGERY

Despite the numerous benefits of neurointerventional surgery, there are attendant risks to these procedures as well. Paramount among these risks is TIA and ischemic strokes caused by thromboemboli from the microcatheters, microguidewires, and devices utilized during the procedure.[9] Qureshi and colleagues conducted a retrospective review of 1,547 patients undergoing coil embolization for intracerebral aneurysm treatment and found that 127 patients (8.2%) experienced thromboembolic events. The vast majority of these events (90.5%) were either TIA or ischemic stroke.[10] In the same study, the authors found that 73 of 834 (8.8%) patients undergoing carotid angioplasty with stent placement also experienced a TIA or ischemic stroke.[10] Similarly, in a meta-analysis of 4,973 patients who underwent intracerebral aneurysm coil embolization, Shapiro et al. documented a thromboembolic complication rate of 8%.[11] Clearly, these thromboembolic events may have serious consequences for patients including hemiparesis, language difficulties, or if severe, even death.

Neuroendovascular surgery has benefited immensely from clinical research involving minimally-invasive techniques used to treat cardiovascular pathologies. Patients suffering from an ST-elevation myocardial infarction (STEMI) may be treated with percutaneous coronary intervention (PCI), which usually involves accessing the coronary vessels remotely through the femoral vessels with recanalization of the diseased coronary vessel and stent placement. The coronary arteries can be dilated by balloon angioplasty and/or various types of stents (e.g., bare metal or drug-eluting stents). Given the high morbidity and mortality from an acute rupture of an atherosclerotic coronary plaque with subsequent stenosis, these stent-assisted revascularization procedures have yielded superior outcomes when compared with medical therapy alone for patients with STEMI.[12-15] However, similar thromboembolic risks exist for patients undergoing PCI that could potentially lead to exacerbation of pre-existing coronary artery stenosis, myocardial infarction, or other end-organ damage caused by thromboemboli. In addition, the risk of coronary stent thrombosis with resulting death or non-fatal MI tends to be unacceptably high without the use of peri- and post-procedural antiplatelet prophylaxis.[16]

Numerous studies in interventional cardiology have analyzed the effects of antiplatelet therapy as a means to counteract the thromboembolic risks of PCI. Initially, aspirin (325 mg PO daily) was utilized as thromboembolic prophylactic monotherapy in patients undergoing PCI. However, increasing evidence soon supported the efficacy of DAPT with clopidogrel in the prevention of thromboembolic catheter-related complications. For example, Mehta et al. retrospectively examined the effects of aspirin and clopidogrel DAPT on thromboembolic events after PCI.[17] In their cohort of 1,313 patients on aspirin and clopidogrel versus 1,345 patients on aspirin alone, they observed a 31% reduction in MI and cardiovascular death in those patients treated with DAPT (169 events in the aspirin only group versus 116 events in the clopidogrel and aspirin group; relative risk = 0.7; p = 0.002).[17] Similar results were seen in the Clopidogrel in Unstable Angina to Prevent Recurrent Ischemic Events (CURE) trial. This study looked at 12,562 patients randomized to either receiving both aspirin and clopidogrel or aspirin and placebo. The primary study endpoints consisted of cardiovascular death, MI, and stroke. Those patients in the DAPT (aspirin and clopidogrel) group were found to have decreased rates of the primary endpoints as compared to those patients treated with aspirin monotherapy, especially in patients undergoing PCI (9.6% in the aspirin and clopidogrel group compared to 13.2% in the aspirin only group; relative risk = 0.72).[18] Other cardiology studies have recapitulated the beneficial effects afforded by peri- and post-procedural DAPT for PCI with large numbers of patients.[18-20] Based largely upon these studies, the American College of Cardiology Foundation and the American Heart Association recommended that patients undergoing PCI should receive clopidogrel (loading dose of 600 mg PO, followed by 75 mg PO daily for at least 12 months) in addition to aspirin following the placement of drug-eluting stents. Furthermore, patients undergoing PCI who receive bare metal stents should have full dose aspirin therapy with 75 mg PO clopidogrel each day for at least one month.[21-22]

Mechanistically, clopidogrel is a thienopyridine antiplatelet agent that inhibits the adenosine diphosphate (ADP) receptor, specifically the $P2Y_{12}$ receptor. The $P2Y_{12}$ receptor is a G-protein coupled receptor that serves to activate platelets by potentiating granule secretion, platelet recruitment, and platelet aggregation.[23] Clopidogrel is a prodrug that requires hepatic transformation for conversion into an active metabolite. That metabolite, in turn, irreversibly binds to and inhibits the $P2Y_{12}$ receptor, thereby preventing platelet activation. Because clopidogrel must be metabolized to its active thiol form in the liver, its anti-platelet effects are not immediately manifested. Given the differing mechanisms of action and pharmacokinetics of clopidogrel and aspirin (the latter being an irreversible, non-specific cyclooxygenase inhibitor that prevents the formation of thromboxane A2), these two agents in concert provide a synergistic inhibitory effect on platelet function.[24]

Despite substantial evidence documenting the safety and efficacy of DAPT for PCI from the cardiology literature, very little evidence exists regarding the use of DAPT in neuroendovascular surgery. In the absence of randomized controlled trials—or even level II evidence from well-designed clinical studies—to guide the administration of antiplatelet agents in neurointerventional surgery, many of the standard treatment paradigms have been extrapolated from the clinical research in other disciplines. Current dosing recommendations include aspirin (325 mg PO daily) and clopidogrel (75 mg PO daily) for seven days prior to a neurointerventional procedure (and at least one month after the procedure) following placement of an intraluminal stent.[9, 25] In the case of newer flow-diverting devices (e.g., PED), antiplatelet may be recommended for a much longer time to prevent untoward vascular occlusion (e.g., 6 months to 1 year).[26] The typical daily dose of clopidogrel (75 mg PO) is commonly started between 3 and 7 days prior to therapy so that the drug can reach therapeutic levels prior to intervention.[27] To achieve even more rapid platelet inhibition, a bolus of 300 mg or 600 mg is administered which usually exerts a biological effect on platelet function within hours. The Clopidogrel for the Reduction of Events During Observation (CREDO) study—a cardiology trial designed to evaluate the efficacy and safety of clopidogrel therapy for one year and the effects of a clopidogrel loading dose prior to elective PCI—showed that a 300 mg oral loading dose given at least 6 hours prior to PCI led to a ~40% reduction in death, MI, or need for urgent revascularization.[20] Even higher loading doses of clopidogrel (600 mg PO) were found to achieve a more rapid effect on platelet dysfunction, exhibit lower rates of antiplatelet resistance, and prevent cardiac death and MI in PCI.[28-30] As a result of these studies, aspirin and clopidogrel DAPT has been recommended for most neuroendovascular procedures.

In general, research on the topic of DAPT in neurointerventional surgery is limited. Some studies however, have examined aspirin and clopidogrel

DAPT in the neurological and neurosurgical patient populations. A study from Yamada et al. retrospectively examined thromboembolic complications of elective intracerebral aneurysm coil embolization when patients were treated with (1) no antiplatelet treatment, (2) antiplatelet therapy following coil embolization, or (3) antiplatelet therapy both before and during coil embolization. Of the 369 patients in the study, they found that symptomatic thromboembolic events occurred in 4 (16.0%) of 25 patients with no antiplatelet drug therapy, 2 (2.3%) of 86 patients receiving post-procedural antiplatelet agents, and in only 5 (1.9%) of 258 patients receiving both pre- and post-procedural antiplatelet therapy ($p = 0.004$ for antiplatelet agent versus no antiplatelet agent) (Table 1). These results were statistically significant, although direct comparisons between treatment groups could not be achieved.[31] This work served to support the hypothesis that antiplatelet therapy was necessary for pre- and post-procedural management of neurointerventional procedures.

Hwang et al. examined the effects of antiplatelet agents on thromboembolic complication rates after elective intracerebral coil embolization. Of the 328 patients retrospectively analyzed, no antiplatelet medications were administered in 95 cases, a single antiplatelet agent (either aspirin or clopidogrel) was used in 61 cases, and DAPT was given in 172 cases. For all cases, antiplatelet agents were given prior to the procedure, with post-procedure antiplatelet therapy reserved for intraoperative thromboembolic complications (mechanical atherosclerotic plaque dislodgement, coil protrusion into the parent artery, or clear thrombus observed on intra-procedural angiography). The authors found 11 (3.4%) cases of thromboembolic events, 6 (6.3%) in the no-treatment group and 5 (2.1%) in the treatment group ($p = 0.085$). Importantly, after performing a subgroup analysis on those cases where multiple microcatheters were used simultaneously, the authors found an overall thromboembolic risk reduction of 85.2% between the no-treatment group and the group receiving antiplatelet agents (12.8% versus 2.1%, respectively; $p = 0.023$) (Table 1). No difference in the incidence of hemorrhagic complications between the groups was noted.[32]

Table 1. Studies assessing thromboembolic complications in neurointerventional procedures with antiplatelet therapy

Study	Treatment groups	n	Outcome measure	# affected	p-value
Yamada, et al.	No antiplatelet agents	25	Thromboembolic complications	4 (16.0%)	0.004 between no-agent and agent groups
	Antiplatelet agents post procedure	86		2 (2.3%)	
	Antiplatelet agents pre and post procedure	258		5 (1.9%)	
Hwang, et al.	No antiplatelet agents	39	Procedural thrombotic event, TIA, stroke within 2 days	5 (12.8%)	0.023 for multiple microcat-heter technique
	Aspirin, clopidogrel, or both	94		2 (2.1%)	
Layton, et al.	No antiplatet agents	144	Thromboembolic complications	12 (8.3%)	0.01 between clopidogre l and non-clopidogre l groups
	DAPT	25		0 (0.0%)	
	ASA only	32		1 (3.1%)	
	Clopidogrel only	7		0 (0.0%)	
Matsumoto, et al.	Aspirin only	69	MRI hyperintensity	27 (39.1%)	0.02
	Clopidogrel 75mg/day for 3 days prior and 1 day after	63		13 (20.6%)	
	Aspirin only	69	Periprocedural thromboembolism	5 (7.2%)	0.3
	Clopidogrel 75mg/day for 3 days prior and 1 day after	63		2 (3.2%)	
Amenta, et al	600mg loading dose clopidogrel, 75mg clopidogrel/81mg aspirin maintainence	65	Intraoperative stent thrombosis	5 (7.7%)	
Rossen, et al.	81mg aspirin/75mg clopidogrel x 6 weeks with 325mg aspirin indefinitely	121	Ischemic events	6 (4.3%)	
Mocco, et al.	Aspirin/clopidogr el DAPT	213	Delayed thromboembolic events	7 (3.0%)	

In their series of 221 patients undergoing coil embolization of intracerebral aneurysms, Layton et al. observed 13 thromboembolic complications; twelve (92.3%) of these complications occurred in patients not taking pre-procedural antiplatelet medications. Further, clopidogrel was found to have a statistically significant effect in reducing thromboembolic events and local thrombus formation ($p = 0.01$) (Table 1).[33] This study underscores the necessity of clopidogrel antiplatelet therapy for reducing untoward thrombotic events in neurointerventional surgery. Matsumoto and colleagues prospectively examined 63 patients receiving clopidogrel therapy alone (75 mg PO daily for 3 days before and 1 day after) for endovascular treatment of unruptured intracerebral aneurysms and compared this group to patients receiving peri-procedural aspirin therapy alone. The authors found that thromboembolic events were lower in the clopidogrel group compared to the aspirin group (3.2% versus 7.2%, respectively), although these results were not statistically significant ($p = 0.3$) (Table 1). They also noted fewer areas of hyperintensity on 24-hour post-procedural diffusion-weighted magnetic resonance imaging in the clopidogrel group as compared to the aspirin group (20.6% versus 39.1%, respectively; $p = 0.02$), thus suggesting a decreased rate of clinical or sub-clinical ischemic strokes.[34] Finally, Amenta et al. observed a thromboembolic complication rate of 7.7% in 65 patients who underwent a neurointerventional procedure and were loaded with clopidogrel (600 mg orally) followed by DAPT maintainence therapy.[50]

Rossen et al. analyzed the effects of discontinuing post-procedural clopidogrel therapy on the rate of thromboembolism in 121 patients who had undergone either stent-assisted aneurysm coil embolization or stent-in-stent flow diversion. They showed that discontinuation of a 6-week clopidogrel treatment regimen resulted in a 5% rate of significant ischemic events (Table 1). This study strongly argues for longer post-procedural treatment times with clopidogrel therapy in the setting of certain neuroendovascular procedures.[35] Meanwhile, Mocco et al. found that in 213 patients treated with stent-assisted coiling for elective intracerebral aneurysms, 3% of patients had delayed thromboembolic events—all of which were associated with premature cessation of post-procedural DAPT.[36]

Taken together, the preponderance of data suggests that the routine use of pre- and post-procedural aspirin and clopidogrel DAPT for neurointerventional surgery has led to a marked reduction in TIA and ischemic strokes. While aspirin monotherapy is more effective than no therapy at all, the combination of aspirin and clopidogrel leads to a greater—and perhaps synergistic—reduction in thromboembolic complications after neurointerventional surgery. Further, the premature discontinuation of clopidogrel therapy may be associated with an increased risk of thromboembolism for certain procedures.

For these cases, post-procedural clopidogrel therapy for greater than 6 weeks is recommended.

Neurologically-Relevant Hemorrhagic Complications of Clopidogrel

Without question, clopidogrel has a preventative role in reducing the rates of peri- and post-procedural thromboembolism in neurointerventional surgery. However, this drug is not without significant hemorrhagic risk. Unlike bleeding into other body compartments that may tolerate a significant volume of blood (e.g., abdomen, pelvis, thorax), even minor amounts of intracerebral hemorrhage can quickly lead to devastating increases in intracranial pressure given the unforgiving confines of the bony calvarium. Moreover, the brain is arguably the most eloquent and exquisitely sensitive human organ, with a poor capacity for tolerating hemorrhagic insults. This makes the decision for antiplatelet therapy even more challenging in this patient population, as the neurointerventionalist oftentimes must balance the morbid equilibrium between hemorrhage and thrombosis.

Numerous studies have demonstrated that antiplatelet therapy—in the setting of both spontaneous intracerebral hemorrhage (ICH) and traumatic brain injury—is an independent predictor of increased morbidity and mortality.[37-41] In their cohort of 90 patients on antiplatelet therapy and 89 patients not on antiplatelet agents who presented with traumatic ICH, Ohm et al. found that patients on antiplatelet agents had a 23% mortality rate as compared to 8.9% in those patients not on antiplatelet agents.[42] In another study, patients on antiplatelet therapy were also more likely to present with higher grade hemorrhage than those not on antiplatelet therapy.[43] Campbell et al. observed that patients with spontaneous ICH on clopidogrel demonstrated increased hematoma expansion, increased in-hospital mortality, and decreased home discharge rates as compared to those on aspirin therapy alone.[44] Another study on traumatic ICH in the elderly population demonstrated a 14-fold increase in the risk of death and 3-fold increase in discharge to long-term rehab in patients on clopidogrel compared to those not on clopidogrel.[45] Gaetani et al. found an increased correlation between traumatic brain injury in elderly patients (age > 70 years) taking antiplatelet therapy and poor outcome.[46] Clopidogrel use has also been implicated in the formation of spontaneous subdural hematoma, requiring extensive reversal before proceeding with burr hole drainage.[47]

Several landmark clinical trials have examined the safety and efficacy of prolonged clopidogrel therapy (with or without aspirin) and have observed a significant rate of spontaneous, life-threatening bleeding complications. The Management of Athero-Thrombosis with Clopidogrel in High-Risk Patients with Recent TIA or Ischemic Stroke (MATCH) study assessed 7,599 patients with prior cerebrovascular ischemic events (stroke or TIA). These patients were then randomized to receive either clopidogrel alone or aspirin-clopidogrel DAPT. While the authors found no difference in ischemic stroke, MI, or vascular death rates, they did discover a significantly higher rate of life-threatening hemorrhage in the DAPT group (2.6%) as compared to the group taking clopidogrel alone (1.3%) over the 18-month study period.[48] Furthermore, the risk of symptomatic ICH was ~0.7% in the clopidogrel only group compared to ~1.1% in the DAPT group while the risk of fatal hemorrhage was ~0.3% in the clopidogrel only group versus ~0.4% in the DAPT group. The results of the MATCH trial are singularly relevant to the neuroendovascular patient population given that the study included only patients with cerebrovascular ischemic disease who were on prolonged DAPT with aspirin and clopidogrel. Their reported rate of 2.6% per year of life-threatening hemorrhage in the DAPT group is a sobering value in light of the prolonged DAPT treatment times frequently required for neurointerventional procedures.

The Clopidogrel for High Atherothrombotic Risk and Ischemic Stablilization, Management, and Avoidance (CHARISMA) study randomly assigned 15,603 patients with cardiovascular disease, or multiple risk factors for vascular disease, to a treatment regimen of either clopidogrel (75 mg PO daily) with low-dose aspirin or low-dose aspirin alone with placebo. While the authors did find a modest—but significant—difference between the two groups for the primary outcome measure (MI, stroke, or death from cardiovascular disease), the study also showed a difference between the two groups in terms of severe bleeding complications ($p = 0.09$) with an increased risk of fatal ICH of 0.33% in the clopidogrel group.[49]

Complications of Clopidogrel in Neurointerventional Surgery

While clopidogrel clearly has a role in preventing peri-procedural thromboembolic complications associated with neurointerventional surgery, the use of this drug is associated with hemorrhagic complications. These bleeding events range from major, life-threatening hemorrhage (including intracerebral hemorrhage or hemodynamically significant gastrointestinal or retroperitoneal bleeding) to minor hemorrhage (including epistaxis and groin site hematomas). To further complicate matters, at times endovascular therapy—with concomitant antiplatelet therapy—is required to treat patients with a pre-existing intracerebral hemorrhagic condition. In these tenuous circumstances, it is difficult to weigh the advantages of thromboembolism reduction against the risks of exacerbating a pre-existing hemorrhage.

Table 2. Studies assessing hemorrhagic complications in neurointerventional procedures with antiplatelet therapy

Study	Treatment groups	n	Outcome measure	# affected	p-value
Akbari, et al.	Aspirin/clopidogrel DAPT	55	Hemorrhagic complications	2 (3.6%)	
Hwang, et al.	No antiplatelet agents	95	Hemorrhagic complications	3 (3.2%)	0.17
	Aspirin, clopid-ogrel, or both	233		7 (3.0%)	
Amenta, et al.	600mg loading dose clopidogrel, 75mg clopidogrel/ 81mg aspirin maintainence	65	Hemorrhage	5 (7.7%)	
Zhang, et al.	300mg aspirin/ 75mg clopidogrel for 3 days prior	9	Delayed intracerebral hemorrhage	2 (22.2%)	0.044
	300mg aspirin/ 300mg clopidogrel loading dose	32		0 (0.0%)	
Yamada, et al.	No antiplatelet agents	25	Extracerebral hemorrhage	0 (0.0%)	> 0.99
	Antiplatelet agents	344		11 (3.2%)	
Goh, et al.	Major hemorrhage	3	Platelet inhibition from clopidogrel	94% platelet inhibition	0.0084
	Minor or no hemorrhage	44		24% platelet inhibition	

Amenta and colleagues examined the safety and efficacy of peri-procedural antiplatelet use in the setting of stent-assisted aneurysm coiling after subarachnoid hemorrhage. In their cohort of 65 patients, these authors observed that 5 (7.7%) had a bleeding complication secondary to antiplatelet therapy and 3 (4.6%) had a fatal hemorrhage (Table 2).[50] In their series of 49 patients who underwent stent-assisted coil embolization of elective cerebral aneurysms (requiring routine antiplatelet therapy for 3 days prior to their procedure), Zhang et al. observed a delayed intracranial hemorrhage rate of 22.2% (Table 2). This rate was significantly greater than a similar group of patients who received loading doses of antiplatelet agents just prior to their procedure (2/9 compared to 0/32 cases; $p = 0.04$) Notably, these authors did not report a difference between the two groups in terms of thromboembolic complications.[51] Finally, Goh et al. conducted a prospective study on clopidogrel hyper-responsiveness (defined as > 72% platelet inhibition as measured by the VerifyNow assay) in patients undergoing elective neurointerventional procedures. They found that in 47 patients, 10 (21.3%) developed major or minor hemorrhagic complications (Table 2). They also noted that percent platelet inhibition was higher in patients with more severe hemorrhagic complications (median 94% inhibition) than those who had minor or no hemorrhage (median 24% inhibition; $p = 0.008$). The 7 clopidogrel hyper-responders in this study experienced a hemorrhagic event rate of 42.8%.[52] These results indicate not only that clopidogrel increases the risk of bleeding complications during and after the procedure, but that this risk is related to the level of platelet inhibition achieved.

Based upon the severity of the clopidogrel-related bleeding complication, cessation of all antiplatelet agents—with or without attempted reversal of the antiplatelet effects of clopidogrel—is sometimes recommended. At many institutions, platelet transfusions still serve as the gold standard for antiplatelet reversal despite the lack of strong evidence to support this treatment paradigm.[37, 53-54] Platelet transfusions have been found in ex vivo studies to restore platelet reactivity.[53] It is thought that since clopidogrel and aspirin bind to platelets irreversibly, platelet transfusions provide the patient with a new supply of uninhibited platelets. However, while platelet transfusion continues to be the primary treatment recommendation for patients with intracerebral hemorrhage on antiplatelet agents, numerous studies have shown that platelet transfusion does not improve mortality.[43, 55] More recently, several reports have suggested other medical alternatives for antiplatelet agent reversal. For instance, Altman et al. observed that recombinant factor VIIa can be used to reverse patients on aspirin and clopidogrel.[56] Desmopressin has also been proposed as a means of reversal, possibly by increasing the release of factor VIII and vWF.[54, 57] Nevertheless, a paucity of data is currently available on the effects of platelet reversal on patient outcomes after intracerebral hemorrhage.

CHALLENGES IN USING CLOPIDOGREL FOR NEUROINTERVENTIONAL SURGERY

Unequivocally, a myriad of challenges exist regarding the use of clopidogrel antiplatelet therapy in neurointerventional surgery. One challenge that has become more widely recognized in recent years pertains to the notion of clopidogrel resistance. It is estimated that approximately 5-30% of patients exhibit hypo-responsiveness to clopidogrel therapy.[58-59] Clopidogrel resistance has been postulated to result from changes in hepatic CYP3A4 enzyme activity, which is responsible for conversion of clopidogrel to an active metabolite.[60] Other possibilities include variable drug absorption, differences in clearance, and $P2Y_{12}$ receptor variability. Irrespective of the mechanism involved, however, patients who are resistant to clopidogrel have been shown to have significantly higher rates of coronary stent thrombosis compared to clopidogrel-responders (8.6% vs 2.3%, respectively; $p < 0.001$).[61] Another study from the cardiology literature demonstrated that the level of clopidogrel response (e.g., degree of clopidogrel-induced platelet dysfunction) directly correlates with decreased risk of 30-day major adverse cardiac events after PCI.[62]

With respect to neurointerventional surgery, Ryu and colleagues examined the effects of antiplatelet resistance in patients undergoing elective intracerebral aneurysm coil embolization. In their cohort of 53 patients, the authors observed a remarkable increase in thromboembolic complications in clopidogrel non-responders as compared to clopidogrel responders. The authors used the VerifyNow assay to assess the effect of aspirin and clopidogrel on platelet function. Platelet inhibition was defined as an aspirin reaction unit (ARU) of greater than 550 for aspirin and a platelet inhibition of less than 40% for clopidogrel. Five patients (9.4%) in their study experienced thromboembolic complications; importantly, all five of these patients demonstrated resistance to both aspirin and clopidogrel as measured by the VerifyNow assay. Patients with a complication had a median aspirin resistance level of 630 ARU versus 468.5 ARU in the group without complication.

Median clopidogrel resistance was 23% in the complication group compared to 35% in the group without complication.[63] The high incidence of clopidogrel hypo-responders in the general population has led endovascular surgeons to more frequently, and diligently, monitor the level of platelet dysfunction prior interventional procedures. In addition, consideration should be given to postponing elective neuroendovascular procedures if the immediate pre-procedural level of platelet function is inappropriately high, or low, in the face of antiplatelet therapy.

A growing body of evidence also suggests that escalating the pre- and/or peri-procedural clopidogrel dose may overcome the hypo-responsiveness seen in most patients. For example, one group demonstrated that by loading patients with 600 mg PO of clopidogrel before the procedure—as opposed to the lower doses typically utilized—the incidence of drug resistance dropped by 22%.[64] Similarly, increasing the daily maintenance dose from 75 to 150 mg PO was shown by one author to markedly lower rates of clopidogrel resistance without precipitating hemorrhagic complications.[65] Neubauer et al. showed that by tailoring clopidogrel treatment regimens to the individual patient (e.g., either by utilizing a higher-dose regimen, repeating the loading dose, doubling the maintenance dose, or employing additional antiplatelet agents) they were able to reduce the incidence of clopidogrel resistance from 23.6% to 5.0%.[66]

The interventional cardiology field recently addressed the import question of whether to escalate antiplatelet therapy in the setting of post-PCI clopidogrel resistance with a large, randomized controlled trial: Gauging Responsiveness with a VerifyNow Assay: Impact on Thrombosis and Safety (GRAVITAS).[67] In this trial, 5429 patients on standard clopidogrel regimens (75 mg PO daily) underwent VerifyNow testing 12-24 hours after PCI. Subsequently, the 2214 (41%) clopidogrel hypo-responders (defined as platelet reactivity units ≥ 230) were randomized to continue their current clopidogrel dose or to receive an additional loading dose (600 mg PO) and escalate their daily maintenance dose (to 150 mg PO). At six months, the primary endpoints (cardiovascular death, MI, and stent thrombosis) were identical between the two groups (2.3%) and bleeding complications were not significantly different these between groups. Notably, most patients enrolled into the study were relatively "low-risk" for future thromboembolic events, with ~80% having stable coronary artery disease. While the results of this trial have been negative to date, it represents the first large study to examine whether optimizing the level of clopidogrel-induced platelet dysfunction alters patient outcomes after interventional surgery. Whether we should translate the results from this interventional cardiology study to assist in the post-procedural management of neuroendovascular surgery patients is currently unclear. Certainly, large differences exist with regard to baseline patient characteristics, specific devices used, disease processes treated, and hemodynamic systems involved (e.g., cerebrovasculature vs. coronary vasculature). In addition, recent literature suggests that pre-procedural levels of DAPT-induced platelet dysfunction—as measured by the VerifyNow assay—may predict major adverse peri-procedural complications in neuroendovascular surgery. In their cohort of 44 patients (undergoing 48 procedures for PED placement for elective, unruptured intracerebral aneurysms), Delgado et al. observed 4 (8.3%) major thromboembolic and hemorrhagic complications. Notably, all major procedural complications occurred in either patients who were considered clopidogrel hypo-responders (PRU value of > 240) and were given additional pre-procedural antiplatelet agents without rescheduling the procedure or in patients considered clopidogrel hyper-responders (PRU value of < 60) shortly before the complication.[68]

Many authorities in the field of neurointerventional surgery are utilizing novel antiplatelet agents in the immediate pre-procedural period to combat the issue of clopidogrel resistance.[69] Recently, the antiplatelet agent prasugrel has been increasingly utilized for both PCI and neurointerventional surgery. Prasugrel is a third generation oral thienopyridine pro-drug that irreversibly inhibits the $P2Y_{12}$ receptor, thereby decreasing platelet aggregation.[70] The drug is rapidly metabolized in both the liver and intestinal mucosa to an active metabolite that has a half-life of approximately 4 hours.[71-72] Prasugrel has the benefit of more potent and rapid inhibition of platelet aggregation as well as decreased response variability.[73-74] The typical dosing of prasugrel is a 60 mg oral loading dose followed by a maintenance dose of 10 mg daily. However, DAPT with aspirin and prasugrel may lead to an increased risk of major hemorrhagic complications as compared to DAPT with aspirin and clopidogrel in both PCI [75-77] and neuroendovascular surgery.[78] Recently, Akbari et al.[78] compared the rate of hemorrhagic complications in those patients undergoing neuroendovascular surgery who were pre-treated with aspirin/clopidogrel DAPT ($n = 55$) or aspirin/prasugrel DAPT ($n = 31$). Notably, those patients who received aspirin/prasugrel DAPT received prasugrel in addition to clopidogrel because of an inadequate response to aspirin/clopidogrel DAPT alone. They observed that 3.6% of patients in the aspirin/clopidogrel group had major hemorrhagic complications compared to 19.4% in the aspirin/prasugrel group ($p = 0.02$). Conversely, Stetler and colleagues [94] found 16 patients who underwent neurointerventional procedures with prasugrel therapy at their institution, none of which had ischemic or hemorrhagic complications. The loading dose used in this study was 40 mg with a mean duration of therapy of 3 months. This study did not compare patients on prasugrel therapy with other antiplatelet agents.

In addition to managing patients with clopidogrel hypo-responsiveness, another significant challenge to the field of neurointerventional surgery is the attenuating effects of other medications—namely, proton pump inhibitors (PPI)—on the platelet response to clopidogrel. Current medical recommendations advocate that all patients on DAPT also receive a PPI in order to minimize the risk of gastrointestinal bleeding (GI) complications.[79] While aspirin therapy alone prevents prostaglandin production within the gastric mucosa thereby predisposing to ulcer formation and GI hemorrhage,[80] the risk of GI bleeding is further increased with aspirin and clopidogrel DAPT.[81] While PPI and H2 blockers lower gastric acidity and facilitate ulcer healing, there has been recent concern that PPI—specifically, omeprazole—interfere with the absorption of antiplatelet agents through their effects on gastric pH and hepatic metabolism.[82] For example, in the randomized double-blinded Omeprazole Clopidogrel Aspirin (OCLA) study, patients who received cardiac stent placement and were placed on aspirin/clopidogrel DAPT with the PPI omeprazole exhibited a significantly decreased clopidogrel inhibitory effect on platelet $P2Y_{12}$ function.[83] The clinical impact of these findings, however, was not addressed in this study. The randomized controlled trial Clopidogrel and the Optimization of Gastrointestinal Events (COGENT) examined the clinical consequences of PPI therapy in patients on DAPT for coronary artery disease with stent placement.[84] Although the study was prematurely halted due to lack of funding, in the > 3,700 patient analyzed omeprazole treatment resulted in a 66% reduction in GI hemorrhage at 6 months with no apparent difference in early adverse cardiac events as compared to patients on DAPT without omeprazole. Major criticisms of the COGENT study abound, however, including disapproval of the patient enrollment criteria and designation of primary cardiac endpoints.[85] The COGENT results were also called into question by a larger, population-based, retrospective cohort study: the Clopidogrel Medco Outcomes Study.[86] In this study of 16,690 patients (9,862 patients taking clopidogrel therapy alone and 6,828 patients taking clopidogrel with a PPI), concomitant use of a PPI was associated with a significantly higher rate of major adverse cardiac events one year after coronary stent placement.[86] Taken together, these studies suggest that patients on DAPT and omeprazole may be at risk for clopidogrel hypo-responsiveness with subsequent adverse events.

In light of these abovementioned studies, many neurointerventional surgeons have assumed a heighted awareness of antiplatelet medication management in those patients taking PPI therapy. Clearly, careful attention should be paid to the level of platelet dysfunction achieved with DAPT in this patient population before any neuroendovascular procedure. In addition, one should have a low threshold for substituting PPI therapies (e.g., replacing omeprazole therapy with an alternative PPI or H2 antagonist), particularly given the recent findings that non-omeprazole PPI seem to have little effect on clopidogrel-induced platelet dysfunction.[82]

METHODS FOR CLOPIDOGREL MONITORING IN NEUROINTERVENTIONAL SURGERY

To determine which patients have appropriately responded to clopidogrel therapy, numerous assays have been developed to assess platelet function. The first of these tests developed—and currently the gold standard assay of platelet function—was platelet aggregometry. In this method, blood is centrifuged to obtain a platelet-rich supernatant. Thereafter, the solution is heated to 37ºC between a light source and a photocell. A platelet agonist, such as ADP, is subsequently added to the platelet-rich solution and the level of aggregation is measured by assessing the optical density of the solution over time.[87] While accurate and reproducible, this test is very expensive, labor-intensive, and not readily available at all institutions. A second widely used test is the Platelet Function Analyzer-100 (PFA). This assay exposes platelets in whole blood with citrate to shear stress in a capillary tube. The flow of the blood through the capillary tube with a membrane of collagen and either ADP or epinephrine is then measured. Eventually, the solution develops a platelet plug and occludes the capillary tube aperture. The time required for tube occlusion is called the closure time. Aspirin increases the closure time when epinephrine is used, while clopidogrel increases the closure time when ADP is used.[88-89] This test is simple, expedient, and is of particular value in testing for von Willebrand disease. However, normalization of platelet function using desmopressin—as measured by the PFA-100—has not been found to reduce peri- and post-operative bleeding events in the neurosurgical patient population.[90] A third test, the VerifyNow-P2Y$_{12}$, is an expedient assay that utilizes a combination of ADP and prostaglandin E1 to directly quantify the effects of clopidogrel on its target receptor (e.g., P2Y12). While prostaglandin E1 attenuates ADP-mediated increases in intracellular calcium via the $P2Y_{12}$ receptor, ADP potentiates platelet activity through its ligand-receptor interactions. This test has the advantage of a superior ability to quantify clopidogrel activity as compared to the PFA-100 assay.[91]

Recently, the Verify Thrombosis Risk Assessment Study (VERITAS) examined platelet responsiveness to clopidogrel therapy in patients with a history of pre-existing vascular disease or multiple risk factors for vascular disease.[92] In this prospective trial, 147 patients underwent VerifyNow platelet function testing (1) before clopidogrel administration and either at (2) 24 hours following a 450 mg PO loading dose or (2) 7 days after chronic daily clopidogrel therapy (75 mg PO). Overall, clopidogrel therapy resulted in a mean reduction in platelet reactivity units of 64.0 ± 25.3%. From these data, the authors concluded that VerifyNow-$P2Y_{12}$ is a fast, reliable, and sensitive assay for the monitoring of platelet dysfunction during clopidogrel therapy. It should be noted, however, that VerifyNow exhibits some intra- and inter-patient variability in platelet aggregation measurements and requires a whole-blood sample.[93]

While the field of interventional surgery has made significant advances toward increasing the sensitivity and specificity of platelet function assays, none of these tests afford consistent, reproducible results when compared against one another.[93] This unfortunate lack of consistency has led many authorities to question whether these assays are appropriate for the clinical quantification of platelet inhibition by clopidogrel. To this end, it remains challenging to directly compare the results of clinical research papers utilizing these different assays. Perhaps a more ubiquitous obstacle regarding clopidogrel-induced platelet dysfunction is the lacking expert consensus of what constitutes a clinically appropriate level of platelet inhibition. For example, in patients undergoing elective neurointerventional surgical procedures requiring DAPT, one author utilized greater than 40% inhibition by VerifyNow[78] as a marker of clopidogrel function, while another employed a metric of greater than 20% inhibition.[94] Further variation exists in the cardiology literature, which has used a range of 32-70% inhibition as cut-offs for responders and non-responders.[95] It is this lack of consistency that makes clinical judgments regarding these assays difficult for neurointerventional surgeons. At our institution, we routinely begin patients on aspirin (325 mg PO daily) and clopidogrel (75 mg PO daily) at least one week prior to their procedure. In the immediate pre-procedural period, the degree of platelet dysfunction is then measured using the VerifyNow assay. We designate clopidogrel responders as those patients with ≥ 30% inhibition of platelet function (e.g., 30-60% platelet inhibition corresponds approximately to PRU values between 214-131, respectively). In cases of clopidogrel hypo- or non-responsiveness, we routinely load patients with prasugrel (60 mg PO once) prior to their procedure and continue this drug for a variable post-procedural period of time (10 mg PO daily). For patients weighing less than 70 kilograms, we typically lower the prasugrel dose (loading: 30 mg PO once; maintenance: 5 mg PO daily). For clopidogrel non-responders requiring additional antiplatelet agents, we closely monitor the post-procedural levels of platelet function using the VerifyNow assay.

Conclusion

Despite the risks and challenges associated with the use of clopidogrel in neurointerventional surgery, aspirin and clopidogrel DAPT remains the current standard for reducing thromboembolic complications. In agreement with these findings, the premature discontinuation of clopidogrel directly correlates with increased thromboembolic events in this patient population. DAPT with aspirin (325 mg PO daily) and clopidogrel (75 mg PO daily for 7 days prior to, and one month following, procedures) is recommended as appropriate thromboembolic prophylaxis for neuroendovascular intervention, whereas a clopidogrel loading dose of 300-600 mg is recommended for urgent intervention. An increasing concern in the field of neurointerventional surgery is the high incidence of patients exhibiting clopidogrel hypo- and hyper-responsiveness, which may precipitate thromboembolic and hemorrhagic complications, respectively. While a myriad of assays exist to measure this phenomenon, no single test affords the sensitivity and specificity necessary for a definitive diagnosis. Also, there is no consensus definition as to what percentage of platelet inhibition constitutes either clopidogrel resistance or an appropriate response to therapy. Amidst the varying paradigms for administering clopidogrel and measuring its effectiveness, more research is clearly required to confidently answer these important questions. One must remember, however, that neurointerventional surgery remains a nascent field and that the rapid evolution of novel therapies frequently outstrips empirical evidence to support their use. We must be cognizant of these challenges as we move forward to further enhance procedural safety and efficacy for our patients.

References

[1] Jeon YI; Kwon do H. Current status and future prospect of endovascular neurosurgery. *J Korean Neurosurg Soc*, 2008, 43(2), 69-78.

[2] Kallmes DF, Ding YH, Dai D, Kadirvel R, Lewis DA, Cloft HJ. A new endoluminal, flow-disrupting device for treatment of saccular aneurysms. *Stroke*, 2007, 38, 2346-2352.

[3] Cekirge HS, Saatci I, Geyik S, Yavuz K, Ozturk H, Pamuk G. Intrasaccular combination of metallic coils and onyx liquid embolic agent for the endovascular treatment of cerebral aneurysms. *J Neurosurg*, 2006, 105, 706-712.

[4] Cekirge HS, Saatci I, Ozturk HM; Cil B, Arat A, Mawad M, et al. Late angiographic and clinical follow-up results of 100 consecutive aneurysms treated with Onyx reconstruction: largest single-center experience. *Neuroradiology*, 2006, 48, 113-126.

[5] van Rooij WJ, Jacobs S, Sluzewski M, van der Pol B, Beute GN, Sprengers ME. Curative embolization of brain arteriovenous malformations with Onyx: Patient selection, embolization technique, and results. *AJNR Am J Neuroradiol*, 2012, 33(7), 1299-1304.

[6] Sehy JV, Holloway WE, Lin SP, Cross DT 3rd, Derdeyn CP, Moran CJ. Improvement in angiographic cerebral vasospasm after intra-arterial verapamil administration. *AJNR Am J Neuroradiol*, 2010, 31(10), 1923-1928.

[7] Jun P, Ko NU, English JD, Dowd CF, Halbach VV, Higashida RT, Lawton MT, Hetts SW. Endovascular treatment of medically refractory cerebral vasospasm following aneurysmal subarachnoid hemorrhage. *AJNR Am J Neuroradiol*, 2010, 31(10), 1911-1916.

[8] McDougall CG, Spetzler RF, Zabramski JM, Partovi S, Hills NK, Nakaji P, Albuquerque FC. The Barrow Ruptured Aneurysm Trial. *J Neurosurg*, 2012, 116(1), 135-144.

[9] Qureshi AI, Luft AR, Sharma M, Guterman LR, Hopkins LN. Prevention and treatment of thromboembolic and ischemic complications associated with endovascular procedures: Part I--Pathophysiological and pharmacological features. *Neurosurgery*, 2000, 46(6), 1344-1359.

[10] Qureshi AI, Luft AR, Sharma M, Guterman LR, Hopkins LN. Prevention and treatment of thromboembolic and ischemic complications associated with endovascular procedures: Part II - Clinical aspects and recommendations. *Neurosurgery*, 2000, 46(6), 1360-1375.

[11] Shapiro M, Babb J, Becske T, Nelson PK. Safety and efficacy of adjunctive balloon remodeling during endovascular treatment of intracranial aneurysms: a literature review. *AJNR Am J Neuroradiol*, 2008, 29(9), 1777-1781.

[12] Davies RF, Goldberg AD, Forman S, Pepine CJ, Knatterud GL, Geller N, Sopko G, Pratt C, Deanfield J, Conti CR. Asymptomatic Cardiac Ischemia Pilot (ACIP) study two-year follow-up: outcomes of patients randomized to initial strategies of medical therapy versus revascularization. *Circulation*, 1997, 95(8), 2037-2043.

[13] Parisi AF, Folland ED, Hartigan P. A comparison of angioplasty with medical therapy in the treatment of single-vessel coronary artery disease. Veterans Affairs ACME Investigators. *N Engl J Med*, 1992, 326(1), 10-16.

[14] Antman EM, Anbe DT, Armstrong PW Bates ER, Green LA, Hand M, Hochman JS, Krumholz HM, Kushner FG, Lamas GA, Mullany CJ, Ornato JP, Pearle DL, Sloan MA, Smith SC Jr. American College of Cardiology: American Heart Association: Canadian Cardiovascular Society. ACC/AHA guidelines for the management of patients with ST-elevation myocardial infarction--executive summary. A report of the American College of Cardiology/American Heart Association Task Force on Practice Guidelines (Writing Committee to revise the 1999 guidelines for the management of patients with acute myocardial infarction). *J Am Coll Cardiol*, 2004, 44(3), 671-719.

[15] Van de Werf F, Bax J, Betriu A, Blomstrom-Lundqvist C, Crea F, Falk V, Filippatos G, Fox K, Huber K, Kastrati A, Rosengren A, Steg PG, Tubaro M, Verheugt F, Weidinger F, Weis M. ESC Committee for Practice Guidelines (CPG). Management of acute myocardial infarction in patients presenting with persistent ST-segment elevation: the Task Force on the Management of ST-Segment Elevation Acute Myocardial Infarction of the European Society of Cardiology. *Eur Heart J*, 2008, 23, 2909-2945.

[16] Teirstein P, Reilly JP. Late stent thrombosis in brachytherapy: the role of long-term antiplatelet therapy. *J Invasive Cardiol*, 2002, 14(3), 109-114.

[17] Mehta SR, Yusuf S, Peters RJ, Bertrand, ME, Lewis BS, Natarajan MK, Malmberg K, Rupprecht H, Zhao F, Chrolavicius S, Copland I, Fox KA. Effects of pretreatment with clopidogrel and aspirin followed by long-term therapy in patients undergoing percutaneous coronary intervention: the PCI-CURE study. *Lancet*, 2001, 358(9281), 527-533.

[18] Fox KA, Mehta SR, Peters R, Zhao F, Lakkis N, Gersh BJ, Yusuf S. Clopidogrel in Unstable angina to prevent Recurrent ischemic Events Trial. Benefits and risks of the combination of clopidogrel and aspirin in patients undergoing surgical revascularization for non-ST-elevation acute coronary syndrome: the Clopidogrel in Unstable angina to prevent Recurrent ischemic Events (CURE) Trial. *Circulation*, 2004, 110(10), 1202-1208.

[19] Wodlinger AM, Pieper JA. The role of clopidogrel in the management of acute coronary syndromes. *Clin Ther*, 2003, 25(8), 2155-2181.

[20] Steinhubl SR, Berger PB, Mann JT 3rd, Fry ET, DeLago A, Wilmer C, Topol EJ. CREDO Investigators. Clopidogrel for the Reduction of Events During Observation. Early and sustained dual oral antiplatelet therapy following percutaneous coronary intervention: a randomized controlled trial. *JAMA*, 2002, 288(19), 2411-2420.

[21] Kushner FG, Hand M, Smith SC Jr., King SB 3rd, Anderson JL, Antman EM, Bailey SR, Bates ER, Blankenship JC, Casey DE Jr., Green LA, Hochman JS, Jacobs AK, Krumholz HM, Morrison DA, Ornato JP, Pearle DL, Peterson ED, Sloan MA, Whitlow PL, Williams DO. 2009 focused updates: ACC/AHA guidelines for the management of patients with ST-elevation myocardial infarction (updating the 2004 guideline and 2007 focused update) and ACC/AHA/SCAI guidelines on percutaneous coronary intervention (updating the 2005 guideline and 2007 focused update) a report of the American College of Cardiology Foundation/American Heart Association Task Force on Practice Guidelines. *J Am Coll Cardiol*, 2009, 54(23), 2205-2241.

[22] George JC, Danagas GD. 2009 Focused updates to guidelines in ST-elevation myocardial infarction and percutaneous coronary intervention: Application to interventional cardiology. *JACC Cardiovasc Interv*, 2009 3(2), 256-258.

[23] Dorsam RT, Kunapuli SP. Central role of the P2Y12 receptor in platelet activation. *J Clin Invest*, 2004, 113(3), 340-345.

[24] Herbert JM, Dol F, Bernat A, Falotico R, Lalé A, Savi P. The antiaggregating and antithrombotic activity of clopidogrel is potentiated by aspirin in several experimental models in the rabbit. *Thromb Haemost*, 1998, 80(3), 512-518.

[25] Howington JU, Hanel RA, Harrigan MR, Levy EI, Guterman LR, Hopkins LN. The Neuroform stent, the first micocatheter-delivered stent for use in the intracranial circulation. *Neurosurgery*, 2004, 54(1), 2-5.

[26] McAuliffe W, Wenderoth JD. Immediate and midterm results following treatment of recently ruptured intracranial aneurysms with the Pipeline embolization device. *AJNR Am J Neuroradiol*, 2012, 2012(33), 3.

[27] Savcic M, Hauert J, Bachmann F, Wyld PJ, Geudelin B, Cariou R. Clopidogrel loading dose regimens: kinetic profile of pharmacodynamic response in healthy subjects. *Semin Thromb Hemost*, 1999, 25(Suppl 2), 15-19.

[28] Lotrionte M, Biondi-Zoccai GG, Agostoni P, Abbate A, Angiolillo DJ, Valgimigli M, Moretti C, Meliga E, Cuisset T, Alessi MC, Montalescot G, Collet JP Di, Sciascio G, Waksman R, Testa L, Sangiorgi G, Laudito A, Trevi GP, Sheiban, I. Meta-analysis appraising high clopidogrel loading in patients undergoing percutaneous coronary intervention. *Am J Cardiol*, 2007, 100(8), 1199-1206.

[29] Montalescot G, Sideris G, Meuleman C, Bal-dit-Sollier C, Lellouche N, Steg PG, Slama M, Milleron O, Collet JP, Henry P, Beygui F, Drouet L, ALBION Trial Investigators. A randomized comparison of high clopidogrel loading doses in patients with non-ST-segment elevation acute coronary syndromes: the ALBION (Assessment of the Best Loading Dose of Clopidogrel to Blunt Platelet Activation, Inflammation and Ongoing Necrosis) trial. *J Am Coll Cardiol*, 2006, 48(5), 931-938.

[30] Cuisset T, Frere C, Quilici J, Morange PE, Nait-Saidi L, Carvajal J, Lehmann A, Lambert M, Bonnet JL, Alessi MC. Benefit of a 600-mg loading dose of clopidogrel on platelet reactivity and clinical outcomes in patients with non-ST-segment elevation acute coronary syndrome undergoing coronary stenting. *J Am Coll Cardiol*, 2006, 48(7), 1339-1345.

[31] Yamada NK, Cross DT 3rd, Pilgram TK, Moran CJ, Derdeyn CP, Dacey RG Jr. Effect of antiplatelet therapy on thromboembolic complications of elective coil embolization of cerebral aneurysms. *AJNR Am J Neuroradiol*, 2007, 28(9), 1778-1782.

[32] Hwang G, Jung C, Park SQ, Kang HS, Lee SH, Oh CW, Chung YS, Han MH, Kwon OK. Thromboembolic complications of elective coil embolization of unruptured aneurysms: the effect of oral antiplatelet preparation on periprocedural thromboembolic complication. *Neurosurgery*, 2010, 67(3), 743-748.

[33] Layton KF, Cloft HJ, Gray LA, Lewis DA, Kallmes DF. Balloon-assisted coiling of intracranial aneurysms: evaluation of local thrombus formation and symptomatic thromboembolic complications. *AJNR Am J Neuroradiol*, 2007, 28(6), 1172-1175.

[34] Matsumoto Y, Kondo R, Matsumori Y, Shimizu H, Takahashi A, Tominaga T. Antiplatelet therapy for prevention of thromboembolic complications associated with coil embolization of unruptured cerebral aneurysms. *Drugs R D*, 2012, 12(1), 1-7.

[35] Rossen JD, Chalouhi N, Wassef SN, Thomas J, Abel TJ, Jabbour PM, Kung DK, Hasan DM. Incidence of cerebral ischemic events after discontinuation of clopidogrel in patients with intracranial aneurysms treated with stent-assisted techniques. *J Neurosurg*, 2012, 117(5), 929-933.

[36] Mocco J, Fargen KM, Albuquerque FC, Bendok BR, Boulos AS, Carpenter JS, Fiorella DJ, Hoh BL, Howington JU, Liebman KM, Natarajan SK, Rai AT, Rodriguez-Mercado R, Siddiqui AH, Snyder KV, Veznedaroglu E, Hopkins LN, Levy EI. Delayed thrombosis or stenosis following enterprise-assisted stent-coiling: is it safe? Midterm results of the interstate collaboration of enterprise stent coiling. *Neurosurgery*, 2011, 69(4), 908-913.

[37] McMillian WD, Rogers FB. Management of prehospital antiplatelet and anticoagulant therapy in traumatic head injury: a review. *J Trauma*, 2009, 66(3), 942-950.

[38] Creutzfeldt CJ, Weinstein JR, Longstreth WT Jr, Becker KJ, McPharlin TO, Tirschwell DL. Prior antiplatelet therapy, platelet infusion therapy, and outcome after intracerebral hemorrhage. *J Stroke Cerebrovasc Dis*, 2009, 18(3), 221-228.

[39] Jones K, Sharp C, Mangram AJ, Dunn EL. The effects of preinjury clopidogrel use on older trauma patients with head injuries. *Am J Surg*, 2006, 192(6), 743-745.

[40] Roquer J, Rodriguez Campello A, Gomis M, Ois A, Puente V, Munteis E. Previous antiplatelet therapy is an independent predictor of 30-day mortality after spontaneous supratentorial intracerebral hemorrhage. *J Neurol*, 2005, 252(4), 412-416.

[41] Toyoda K, Okada Y, Minematsu K, Kamouchi M, Fujimoto S, Ibayashi S, Inoue, T. Antiplatelet therapy contributes to acute deterioration of intracerebral hemorrhage. *Neurology*, 2005, 65(7), 1000-1004.

[42] Ohm C, Mina A, Howells G, Bair H, Bendick P. Effects of antiplatelet agents on outcomes for elderly patients with traumatic intracranial hemorrhage. *J Trauma*, 2005, 58(3), 518-522.

[43] Ivascu FA, Howells GA, Junn FS, Bair HA, Bendick PJ, Janczyk RJ. Predictors of mortality in trauma patients with intracranial hemorrhage on preinjury aspirin or clopidogrel. *J Trauma*, 2008, 65(4), 785-788.

[44] Campbell PG, Yadla S, Sen AN, Jallo J, Jabbour P. Emergency reversal of clopidogrel in the setting of spontaneous intracerebral hemorrhage. *World Neurosurg*, 2011, 76(1-2), 100-104.

[45] Wong DK, Lurie F, Wong LL. The effects of clopidogrel on elderly traumatic brain injured patients. *J Trauma,* 2008, 65(6), 1303-1308.

[46] Gaetani P, Revay M, Sciacca S, Pessina F, Aimar E, Levi D, Morenghi E. Traumatic brain injury in the elderly: considerations in a series of 103 patients older than 70. *J Neurosurg Sci*, 2012, 56(3),231-237.

[47] Vuk A, Stancic V, Rincić G, Ledinsky M, Grbac L, Stancić N. Nontraumatic bilateral subdural hematoma caused by antiaggregation therapy: case report and review of the literature. *Acta Clin Croat*, 2010, 49(2), 163-168.

[48] Diener HC, Bogousslavsky J, Brass LM, Cimminiello C, Csiba L, Kaste M, Leys D, Matias-Guiu J, Rupprecht HJ. MATCH investigators. Aspirin and clopidogrel compared with clopidogrel alone after recent ischaemic stroke or transient ischaemic attack in high-risk patients (MATCH): randomised, double-blind, placebo-controlled trial. *Lancet*, 2004, 364(9431), 331-337.

[49] Bhatt DL, Fox KA, Hacke W, Berger PB, Black HR, Boden WE, Cacoub P, Cohen EA, Creager MA, Easton JD, Flather MD, Haffner SM, Hamm CW, Hankey GJ, Johnston SC, Mak KH, Mas JL, Montalescot G, Pearson TA, Steg PG, Steinhubl SR, Weber MA, Brennan DM, Fabry-Ribaudo L, Booth J, Topol EJ. CHARISMA Investigators. Clopidogrel and aspirin versus aspirin alone for the prevention of atherothrombotic events. *N Engl J Med*, 2006, 354(16), 1706-1717.

[50] Amenta PS, Dalyai RT, Kung D, Toporowski A, Chandela S, Hasan D, Gonzalez LF, Dumont AS, Tjoumakaris SI, Rosenwasser RH, Maltenfort MG, Jabbour PM. Stent-assisted coiling of wide-necked aneurysms in the setting of acute subarachnoid hemorrhage: experience in 65 patients. *Neurosurgery*, 2012, 70(6), 1415-1429.

[51] Zhang XD, Wu HT, Zhu J, He ZH, Chai WN, Sun XC. Delayed intracranial hemorrhage associated with antiplatelet therapy in stent-assisted coil embolized cerebral aneurysms. *Acta Neurochir Suppl*, 2011, 110, 133-139.

[52] Goh C, Churiloy L, Mitchell P, Dowling R, Yan B. Clopidogrel Hyper-Response and Bleeding Risk in Neurointerventional Procedures. *AJNR Am J Neuroradiol*, 2012, Epub ahead of print.

[53] Vilahur G, Choi BG, Zafar MU, Viles-Gonzalez JF, Vorchheimer DA, Fuster V, Badimon JJ. Normalization of platelet reactivity in clopidogrel-treated subjects. *J Thromb Haemost,* 2007, 5(1), 82-90.

[54] Beshay JE, Morgan H, Madden C, Yu W, Sarode R. Emergency reversal of anticoagulation and antiplatelet therapies in neurosurgical patients. *J Neurosurg*, 2010, 112(2), 307-318.

[55] Ducruet AF, Hickman ZL, Zacharia BE, Grobelny BT, DeRosa PA, Landes E, Lei S, Khandji J, Gutbrod S, Connolly ES Jr. Impact of platelet transfusion on hematoma expansion in patients receiving antiplatelet agents before intracerebral hemorrhage. *Neurol Res*, 2010, 32(7), 706-710.

[56] Altman R, Scazziota A, Delh M, Gonzalez C. Recombinant factor VIIa reverses the inhibitory effect of aspirin or aspirin plus clopidogrel on in vitro thrombin generation. *J Thromb Haemost*, 2006, 4, 2022-2027.

[57] Mannucci PM. Desmopressin (DDAVP) in the treatment of bleeding disorders: the first 20 years. *Blood*, 1997, 90(7), 2515-2521.

[58] Serebruany VL, Steinhubl SR, Berger PB, Malinin AI, Bhatt DL, Topol EJ. Variability in platelet responsiveness to clopidogrel among 544 individuals. *J Am Coll Cardiol*, 2005, 45(2), 246-251.

[59] Gurbel PA, Bliden KP, Hiatt BL, O'Connor CM. Clopidogrel for Coronary Stenting: Response Variability, Drug Resistance, and the Effect of Pretreatment Platelet Reactivity. *Circulation*, 2003, 107(23), 2908-2913.

[60] Lau WC, Grubel PA, Watkins PB, Neer CJ, Hopp AS, Carville DG, Guyer KE, Tait AR, Bates ER. Contribution of hepatic cytochrome P450 3A4 metabolic activity to the phenomenon of clopidogrel resistance. *Circulation*, 2004, 109(2), 166-171.

[61] Buonamici P, Marcucci R, Migliorini A, Gensini GF, Santini A, Paniccia R, Moschi G, Gori AM, Abbate R, Antoniucci D. Impact of platelet reactivity after clopidogrel administration on drug-eluting stent thrombosis. *J Am Coll Cardiol*, 2007, 49(24), 2312-2317.

[62] Hochholzer W, Trenk D, Bestehorn HP, Fischer B, Valina CM, Ferenc M, Gick M, Caputo A, Büttner HJ, Neumann FJ. Impact of the degree of peri-interventional platelet inhibition after loading with clopidogrel on early clinical outcome of elective coronary stent placement. *J Am Coll Cardiol*, 2006, 48(9), 1742-1750.

[63] Ryu DS, Hong CK, Sim YS, Kim CH, Jung JY, Joo JY. Anti-platelet drug resistance in the prediction of thromboembolic complications after neurointervention. *J Korean Neurosurg Soc*, 2010, 48(4), 319-324.

[64] Gurbel PA, Bliden KP, Hayes KM, Yoho JA, Herzog WR, Tantry US. The relation of dosing to clopidogrel responsiveness and the incidence of high post-treatment platelet aggregation in patients undergoing coronary stenting. *J Am Coll Cardiol*, 2005, 45(9), 1392-1396.

[65] Aleil B, Jacquemin L, De Poli F, Zaehringer M, Collet JP, Montalescot G, Cazenave JP, Dickele MC, Monassier JP, Gachet C. Clopidogrel 150 mg/day to Overcome Low Responsiveness in Patients Undergoing Elective Percutaneous Coronary InterventionResults From the VASP-02 (Vasodilator-Stimulated Phosphoprotein-02) Randomized Study. *JACC: Cardiovasc Interv*, 2008, 1(6), 631-638.

[66] Neubauer H, Lask S, Engelhardt A, Mugge A. How to optimise clopidogrel therapy? Reducing the low-response incidence by aggregometry-guided therapy modification. *Thromb Haemost*, 2008, 99(2), 357.

[67] Price MJ, Berger PB, Teirstein PS, Tanguay JF, Angiolillo DJ, Spriggs D, Puri S, Robbins M, Garratt KN, Bertrand OF, Stillabower ME, Aragon JR, Kandzari DE, Stinis CT, Lee MS, Manoukian SV, Cannon CP, Schork NJ, Topol EJ; GRAVITAS Investigators. Standard-vs High-Dose Clopidogrel Based on Platelet Function Testing After Percutaneous Coronary Intervention The GRAVITAS Randomized Trial. *JAMA*, 2011, 305(11), 1097-1105.

[68] Delgado Almandoz JE, Crandall BM, Scholz JM, Fease JL, Anderson RE, Kadkhodayan Y, Tubman DE. Pre-procedure P2Y12 reaction units value predicts perioperative thromboembolic and hemorrhagic complications in patients with cerebral aneurysms treated with the Pipeline Embolization Device. *J neurointerv surg*, 2013.

[69] Angiolillo DJ, Ferreiro JL. Platelet adenosine diphosphate P2Y12 receptor antagonism: Benefits and limitations of current treatment strategies and future directions. *Rev Esp Cardiol*, 2010, 63, 60-76.

[70] Niitsu Y, Jakubowski JA, Sugidachi A, Asai F. Pharmacology of CS-747 (prasugrel, LY640315), a novel, potent antiplatelet agent with in vivo P2Y12 receptor antagonist activity. *Semin Thromb Hemost*, 2005, 31(2),
184-194.

[71] Dobesh PP. Pharmacokinetics and pharmacodynamics of prasugrel, a thienopyridine P2Y12 inhibitor. *Pharmacotherapy*, 2009, 29(9), 1089-1102.

[72] Hagihara K, Kazui M, Ikenaga H, Nanba T, Fusegawa K, Izumi T, Ikeda T, Kurihara A. The intestine as an important contributor to prasugrel

active metabolite formation in vivo. *Drug metab dispos*, 2011, 39(4), 565-570.

[73] Weerakkody GJ, Jakubowski JA, Brandt JT, Farid NA, Payne CD, Zhu J, Warner MR, Naganuma H, Winters KJ. Comparison of speed of onset of platelet inhibition after loading doses of clopidogrel versus prasugrel in healthy volunteers and correlation with responder status. *Am J Cardiol*, 2007, 100(2), 331-336.

[74] Farid NA, Smith RL, Gillespie TA, Rash TJ, Blair PE, Kurihara A, Goldberg MJ. The disposition of prasugrel, a novel thienopyridine, in humans. *Drug Metab Dispos*, 2007, 35(7), 1096-1104.

[75] Wiviott SD, Braunwald E, McCabe CH, Horvath I, Keltai M, Herrman JP, Van de Werf F, Downey WE, Scirica BM, Murphy SA, Antman EM; TRITON-TIMI 38 Investigators. Intensive oral antiplatelet therapy for reduction of ischaemic events including stent thrombosis in patients with acute coronary syndromes treated with percutaneous coronary intervention and stenting in the TRITON-TIMI 38 trial: a subanalysis of a randomised trial. *Lancet*, 2008, 371(9621), 1353-1363.

[76] Armero S, Bonello L, Berbis J, Camoin-Jau L, Lemesle G, Jacquin L, Bonello-Burignat C, Pansieri M, Collet F, Ostorero M, Dignat-George F, Paganelli F. Rate of nuisance bleedings and impact on compliance to prasugrel in acute coronary syndromes. *Am J Cardiol*, 2011, 108(12), 1710-1713.

[77] Wiviott SD, Braunwald E, McCabe CH, Montalescot G, Ruzyllo W, Gottlieb S, Neumann FJ, Ardissino D, De Servi S, Murphy SA, Riesmeyer J, Weerakkody G, Gibson CM, Antman EM; TRITON-TIMI 38 Investigators. Prasugrel versus clopidogrel in patients with acute coronary syndromes. *N Engl J Med*, 2007, 357(20), 2001-2015.

[78] Akbari SH, Reynolds MR, Kadkhodayan Y, Cross DT 3rd, Moran CJ. Hemorrhagic complications after prasugrel (Effient) therapy for vascular neurointerventional procedures. *J Neurointerv Surg*, 2012, [Epub ahead of print].

[79] Bhatt DL, Scheiman J, Abraham NS, Antman EM, Chan FK, Furberg CD, Johnson DA, Mahaffey KW, Quigley EM, Harrington RA, Bates ER, Bridges CR, Eisenberg MJ, Ferrari VA, Hlatky MA, Kaul S, Lindner JR, Moliterno DJ, Mukherjee D, Schofield RS, Rosenson RS, Stein JH, Weitz HH, Wesley DJ; American College of Cardiology Foundation; American College of Gastroenterology; American Heart Association. ACCF/ACG/AHA 2008 Expert Consensus Document on Reducing the Gastrointestinal Risks of Antiplatelet Therapy and NSAID

UseA Report of the American College of Cardiology Foundation Task Force on Clinical Expert Consensus Documents. *J Am Coll Cardiol*, 2008, 52(18), 1502-1517.

[80] García Rodríguez LA, Lin KJ, Hernández-Díaz S, Johansson S. Risk of Upper Gastrointestinal Bleeding With Low-Dose Acetylsalicylic Acid Alone and in Combination With Clopidogrel and Other Medications Clinical Perspective. *Circulation*, 2011, 123(10), 1108-1115.

[81] Moukarbel GV, Signorovitch JE, Pfeffer MA, McMurray JJ, White HD, Maggioni AP, Velazquez EJ, Califf RM, Scheiman JM, Solomon SD. Gastrointestinal bleeding in high risk survivors of myocardial infarction: the VALIANT Trial. *Eur Heart J*, 2009, 30(18), 2226-2232.

[82] Sibbing D, Morath T, Stegherr J, Braun S, Vogt W, Hadamitzky M, Schömig A, Kastrati A, von Beckerath N.. Impact of proton pump inhibitors on the antiplatelet effects of clopidogrel. *Thromb Haemost*, 2009, 101(4), 714-719.

[83] Gilard M, Arnaud B, Cornily JC, Le Gal G, Lacut K, Le Calvez G, Mansourati J, Mottier D, Abgrall JF, Boschat J. Influence of Omeprazole on the Antiplatelet Action of Clopidogrel Associated With AspirinThe Randomized, Double-Blind OCLA (Omeprazole CLopidogrel Aspirin) Study. *J Am Coll Cardiol.*, 2008, 51(3), 256-260.

[84] Bhatt DL, Cryer BL, Contant CF, Cohen M, Lanas A, Schnitzer TJ, Shook TL, Lapuerta P, Goldsmith MA, Laine L, Scirica BM, Murphy SA, Cannon CP; COGENT Investigators. Clopidogrel with or without omeprazole in coronary artery disease. *N Engl J Med*, 2010, 363(20), 1909-1917.

[85] Southworth MR, Temple R. Interaction of clopidogrel and omeprazole. *N Engl J Med*, 2010, 363(20), 1977.

[86] Kreutz RP, Stanek EJ, Aubert R, Yao J, Breall JA, Desta Z, Skaar TC, Teagarden JR, Frueh FW, Epstein RS, Flockhart DA. Impact of proton pump inhibitors on the effectiveness of clopidogrel after coronary stent placement: the clopidogrel medco outcomes study. *Pharmacotherapy*, 2010, 30(8), 787-796.

[87] Michelson, AD. Platelet function testing in cardiovascular diseases. *Circulation*, 2004, 110, 489-493.

[88] Kundu SK, Heilmann EJ, Sio R, Garcia C, Davidson RM, Ostgaard RA. Description of an in vitro platelet function analyzer--PFA-100. *Semin Thromb Hemost*, 1995, 21(Suppl 2), 106-112.

[89] Kratzer MA, Born GV. Simulation of primary hemostasis in vitro. *Hemostasis*, 1985, 5, 357-362.

[90] Karger R, Reuter K, Rohlfs J, Nimsky C, Sure U, Kretschmer V. The Platelet Function Analyzer (PFA-100) as a Screening Tool in Neurosurgery. *ISRN Hematol*, 2012, Epub 2012 Aug 8.

[91] Bouman HJ, Parlak E, van Werkum JW, Breet NJ, ten Cate H, Hackeng CM, ten Berg JM, Taubert D. Which platelet function test is suitable to monitor clopidogrel responsiveness? A pharmacokinetic analysis on the active metabolite of clopidogrel. *J Thromb Haemost*, 2010, 8(3), 482-488.

[92] Malinin A, Pokov A, Spergling M, Defranco A, Schwartz K, Schwartz D, Mahmud E, Atar D, Serebruany V. Monitoring platelet inhibition after clopidogrel with the VerifyNow-P2Y12(R) rapid analyzer: the VERIfy Thrombosis risk ASsessment (VERITAS) study. *Thromb Res*, 2007, 119(3), 277-284.

[93] Lordkipanidzé M, Pharand C, Nguyen TA, Schampaert E, Palisaitis DA, Diodati JG. Comparison of four tests to assess inhibition of platelet function by clopidogrel in stable coronary artery disease patients. *Eur Heart J*, 2008, 29(23), 2877-2885.

[94] Stetler WR, Chaudhary N, Thompson BG, Gemmete JJ, Maher CO, Pandey AS. Prasugrel is effective and safe for neurointerventional procedures. *J Neurointerv Surg*, 2012, Epub ahead of print.

[95] Combescure C, Fontana P, Mallouk N, Berdague P, Labruyere C, Barazer I, Gris JC, Laporte S, Fabbro-Peray P, Reny JL; CLOpidogrel and Vascular ISchemic Events Meta-analysis Study Group. Clinical implications of clopidogrel non-response in cardiovascular patients: a systematic review and meta-analysis. *J Thromb Haemost*, 2010, 8(5), 923-933.

In: Clopidogrel
Editors: J. P. Alesci and A. Victorino
ISBN: 978-1-62948-336-8
© 2014 Nova Science Publishers, Inc.

Chapter 3

CLOPIDOGREL PHARMACOKINETIC: REVIEW OF EARLY STUDIES AND NOVEL EXPERIMENTAL RESULTS

L. Silvestro,[1,*] S. N. Savu,[2,3,#] S. Rizea Savu[1,†] and I. Tarcomnicu[4,‡]

[1]3S-Pharmacological Consultation and Research GmbH, Harpstedt, Germany
[2]University of Medicine and Pharmacy "Carol Davila," Faculty of Pharmacy, Department of Drug, Physical Chemistry and Biopharmacy, Bucharest, Romania
[3]3S-Pharmacological Consultation and Res. SRL. Bucharest, Romania
[4]Pharma Serv International SRL. Bucharest, Romania

* Corresponding author: L. Silvestro, 3S-Pharmacological Consultation and Research GmbH, Koenigsbergerstrasse 1, 27243 Harpstedt, Germany. E-mail: Dreispharmasl@aol.com.

S. N. Savu: University of Medicine and Pharmacy "Carol Davila", Faculty of Pharmacy, Department of Drug Physical Chemistry and Biopharmacy, 6 Traian Vuia Street, 2nd District, 020956 Bucharest, Romania. 3S-Pharmacological Consultation and Res. SRL. 52 Sabinelor Street, 5th District, 050853 Bucharest, Romania.

† S. Rizea Savu: 3S-Pharmacological Consultation and Research GmbH, Koenigsbergerstrasse 1, 27243 Harpstedt, Germany.

‡ I. Tarcomnicu: Pharma Serv International SRL. 52 Sabinelor Street, 5th District, 050853 Bucharest, Romania.

Abstract

In 1998 the European Commission granted the first marketing authorization for the potent anti-platelet aggregation agent clopidogrel to Sanofi Pharma Bristol-Myers Squibb SNC; the pharmacokinetic section of the Scientific Discussion which was part of the European Public Assessment Report stated that plasma levels of the parent compound beyond 2 hours from administration are very low, below the quantification limit of the existing method, and the only pharmacokinetic information available were on the inactive clopidogrel carboxylic metabolite. Clopidogrel appeared from the beginning to be a prodrug; however, detailed information on the chemical structure and pharmacology of the active moiety, the thiol metabolite responsible of the therapeutic action, were only published in 2000 by Savi et al., leaving in any case open the discussion on the pharmacokinetic aspects of this molecule. Four years later, in 2004, Lainesse et al. presented the first clopidogrel pharmacokinetic data in man and, in the same year, Taubert et al. published the first paper on the determination of clopidogrel active metabolite in plasma. It is noteworthy that for many years the analytical methods aiming to quantify clopidogrel in human plasma have encountered big problems. Until in 2010, a more clear understanding of the problem was reached, discovering that a new metabolite of clopidogrel is responsible for back-conversion to clopidogrel during sample handling (Silvestro et al., 2010). In the same years the oxidative steps involved in the synthesis of the active metabolite were studied and cytochrome P450 isoenzymes 2B6, 3A4, 1A1, 1A2 and 2C19 were identified as the most important. As a result of these findings, and of several PK/PD and genotype studies, in 2010, the FDA approved a new label for clopidogrel with a "boxed warning" about the diminished effectiveness of the drug in patients with impaired ability to convert the prodrug into its active form. Meanwhile a lot of progress was done also in the identification and quantitation of other clopidogrel metabolites like oxo-clopidogrel and clopidogrel acyl-glucuronide. Despite 15 years are passed from the introduction of clopidogrel in the market, the pharmacokinetic of this molecule still intrigues and attracts the attention of the scientific community.

1. Introduction

Clopidogrel, as already known from the available literature, is an oral thienopyridine derivative, used as anti-platelet aggregation agent to inhibit blood clots formation in coronary artery diseases, peripheral vascular diseases, and cerebrovascular diseases (SmPC (Summary of Product Characteristics) of Plavix, revised 26 July 2013). Clopidogrel is a prodrug that is absorbed in the intestine and activated in the liver. The conversion of clopidogrel to its active metabolite requires two sequential steps: it is first oxydized to 2-2-oxo-clopidogrel (intermediate metabolite) and subsequently metabolized to the active metabolite through a reaction mediated by multiple P450 cytochromes.

The metabolite exerts its pharmacodynamic action by selectively inhibiting the binding of adenosine diphosphate (ADP) to its platelet $P2Y_{12}$ receptor and the subsequent ADP-mediated activation of the glycoprotein GPIIb/IIIa complex, thereby inhibiting platelet aggregation. Due to the irreversible binding, platelets exposed are affected for the remainder of their lifespan (approximately 7-10 days).

Although a large number of publications provide useful information on clopidogrel, some particularities relating to its pharmacokinetic and pharmacodynamic behavior as well as the sources of the observed intra-individual variability with respect to therapeutic efficacy remain open for debate.

The purpose of this chapter is to provide a comprehensive image of what was thought to be known about clopidogrel pharmacokinetic at the time of the marketing authorization, the new information gathered so far and the aspects that still need further clarifying in the future.

The European Commission granted a marketing authorization valid throughout the European Union for Plavix (clopidogrel) to Sanofi Pharma Bristol-Myers Squibb SNC on 15 July 1998. The pharmacokinetic section of the Scientific Discussion which was part of the EPAR (European Public Assessment Report) of Plavix stated that plasma levels of the parent compound beyond 2 hours from administration are very low and below the quantification limit (0.00025 mg/L) of the existing method, and that the active metabolite, a thiol derivative, was formed by oxidation of clopidogrel to 2-oxo-clopidogrel and subsequent hydrolysis.

The oxidative step was thought to be regulated primarily by the Cytochrome P450 isoenzymes 2B6 and 3A4 and to a lesser extent by 1A1, 1A2 and 2C19 (EMA Scientific Discussion on Plavix, first published 24.10. 2006).

The active thiol metabolite, isolated in vitro, could not be detected in plasma at that time. Detailed information on the chemical structure and pharmacological activity of the active metabolite were published in 2000 by Savi et al., leaving in any case open the discussion on the pharmacokinetic behavioral aspects of this molecule.

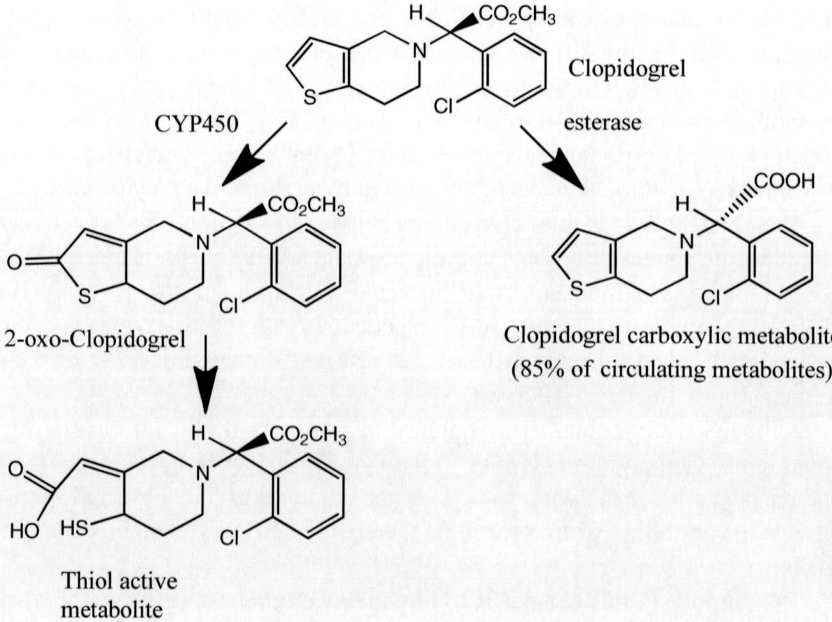

Figure 1. Clopidogrel metabolic pathway according to SmPC.

The known metabolic pathway of clopidogrel, as stated in the SmPC and presented in figure 1, is simple having two directions: on one hand, a desesterification to clopidogrel carboxylic acid, and on the other hand, an oxidation to 2-oxo-clopiopgrel, which undergoes a further oxidation leading to the active metabolite (Figure 1).

Suitable quantification assays were at the time only available for the main circulating inactive metabolite, the carboxylic acid derivative of clopidogrel, which represents about 85% of the circulating compound in plasma; though useful as a marker of absorption, it was admitted that the relevance of conventional pharmacokinetic studies of the inactive metabolite was limited. Thus, many aspects of clopidogrel behavior in special populations or potential interactions with other drugs were studied using dynamic markers such as inhibition of ADP-induced platelet aggregation and prolongation of bleeding time. In the years later, thanks to the improvement in liquid-chromatography-mass spectrometry (HPLC-MS/MS) techniques, methods were successfully developed to determine the parent molecule, clopidogrel, in biological samples of subjects treated with clopidogrel at therapeutic dosage. It is noteworthy to mention here the work performed by Lainesse et al. in 2004.

Still, it was evident that a main open issue for PK/PD studies was the fact that clopidogrel itself is inactive, and the determination of its active metabolite was expected to be much more revealing. Also in 2004, Taubert et al. published the first paper on the determination of clopidogrel active metabolite in plasma. Because a pure synthetic standard of active metabolite was unavailable, the authors based the quantitative evaluation on a surrogate calibration curve of clopidogrel.

Despite this shortcoming the work of the German group was quite a milestone and presented interesting observations also on PK/PD correlation. In 2006 Nirogi et al. published another interesting work comparing the PK of clopidogrel administered in fasting and fed conditions, showing a relevant food effect that was not observed, as reported in the Plavix SmPC, in studies employing a PD approach.

The group of Takahasi et al. described in 2008 the first quantitative method for the determination of clopidogrel active metabolite in plasma using an adequate analytical standard; the method employs a derivatization procedure just upon sampling to minimize the degradation of the metabolite, problem already discussed by Taubert group that also developed and patented (Bundesrepublik Deutschland Deutsches Patent DE 102004046159A1; 2006) a complex procedure to stabilize the samples.

Several other publications presented studies on clopidogrel PK and large variations of C_{max} and $AUC_{0\text{-}t}$ have been observed with the same dose administered. The scientific community raised concerns regarding overestimation of the quantitative results, due to back-conversion of some clopidogrel metabolites into the parent compound.

As a consequence, regulatory authorities were forced to take position on this issue, as it can be seen in EMA's "Questions and Answers: Positions on specific questions addressed to the pharmacokinetics working party" (EMA/ 618604/2008).

According to this paper, the fact that plasma levels of clopidogrel carboxylic acid observed in patients or healthy volunteers treated with clopidogrel are 3 orders of magnitude higher than those of clopidogrel, only a minimum back-conversion of this metabolite could potentially lead to a huge overestimation of clopidogrel plasma levels and would bias the outcome of bioequivalence studies. It was therefore concluded by EMA experts, that clopidogrel bioanalytical method validations should include a demonstration that there is no back-conversion of the major metabolite to the parent drug clopidogrel under all conditions of sample handling (including extraction procedures) and storage.

However, a few publications pointed out that a clopidogrel metabolite, other than carboxylic acid, is the source of back-conversion (Yerino et al. (2006), Garofolo et al. (2009), Silvestro et al. (2010)). The studies carried out by our group showed that clopidogrel acyl glucuronide, rather than oxo-clopidogrel or the active metabolite, is responsible for the back-conversion of clopidogrel (Silvestro et al. (2011)); more information on this aspect, along with representative results are presented in the section regarding analytical issues in clopidogrel determination from plasma.

Along with the analytical advances made over the past years, a great effort has been also oriented to better understand the metabolic pathway of clopidogrel, with emphasys on the identification of markers that can be associated with individual pharmcodynamic variability through genotyping.

In-vitro tests carried out by Kazui et al. (2010) using cDNA-expressed human P450 isoforms have shown that clopidogrel is metabolized to 2-oxo-clopidogrel, the immediate precursor of its pharmacologically active metabolite, in a reaction catalyzed by CYP1A2, CYP2B6 and CYP2C19 with an individual contribution to the formation of 2-oxo-clopidogrel of 35.8, 19.4 and respectively 44.9%. In the same system using 2-oxo-clopidogrel as substrate, detection of the active metabolite of clopidogrel required the addition of glutathione to the system. CYP2B6, CYP2C9, CYP2C19 and CYP3A4 contributed to the production of the active metabolite and their individual contribution was found to be 32.9, 6.76, 20.6 and respectively 39.8%. The studies showed that CYP2C19 contributed substantially to both oxidative steps required in the formation of clopidogrel active metabolite and that CYP3A4 contributed significantly to the second oxidative step and helped explaining the role of genetic polymorphism of CYP2C19 and also the effect of potent CYP3A inhibitors on the pharmacokinetics and pharmacodynamics of clopidogrel. To date, the reduced-function genetic variants in the hepatic cytochrome CYP2C19 gene have been identified as the most prominent contributors to the variability of clopidogrel. As a result of these findings, as well of other studies, in March 12, 2010, FDA approved a new label for clopidogrel with a "boxed warning" about the diminished effectiveness of the drug in patients with impaired ability to convert the drug into its active form. The boxed warning is based on the concern that the anti-platelet aggregation effect of clopidogrel depends primarily on its activation by the cytochrome P450 (CYP) system. Patients with decreased CYP2C19 function because of genetic polymorphisms metabolize clopidogrel poorly and have higher rates of cardiovascular events after acute coronary syndrome (ACS) and percutaneous coronary interventions (PCIs) than patients with normal CYP2C19 function.

The warning also notes that tests are available to identify patients with genetic polymorphisms, and that alternative treatment strategies should be considered in poor metabolizers of the drug (Holmes et al. (2010)).

It is interesting to observe that despite the huge improvement in the analytics of clopidogrel and its metabolites, no work has been published on therapeutic drug monitoring of clopidogrel and only scarce PK data, beside method development, is available for the active metabolite of clopidogrel.

2. Pharmacokinetics of Clopidogrel Carboxylic Acid and Clopidogrel

In the early phase development of clopidogrel, modest analytical sensitivity was a major issue for quantitative measurements in biological samples. As aforementioned, plasma levels of the parent drug were considered below the limit of detection of most methods; therefore bioavailability studies have been conducted first using the major inactive metabolite, clopidogrel carboxylic acid *(SR26334)*, as main parameter.

Back in 1998, Lagorce et al. published for the first time information about plasma concentrations of SR26334.The authors used GC-MS as analytical technique and the sample preparation protocol was quite complex, involving liquid-liquid extraction followed by solid-phase extraction and derivatization with *n*-ethyl diisopropyl-ethylamine and α-bromo-2,3,4,5,6-pentafluoro toluene.

Table 1 resumes the PK data measured in published papers up to date and also data available from studies of our group.

All authors describe quantification methods based on HPLC-MS/MS, except Lagorce (1998) employing GC-MS and Yousef et al. (2013) using liquid chromatography with UV detection. Von Beckenrath et al. (2005) developed and validated a method for simultaneous determination of clopidogrel, its carboxylic acid metabolite (SR26334) and its active thiol metabolite (the later on a surrogate curve of clopidogrel) on a Kromasil C8 column, using 1-methyl-4-phenylpyridinium bromide as internal standard. Ksycinska et al. (2006) validated on Luna C18 column a method only for the quantification of the carboxylic acid, repaglinide being the internal standard. Two studies performed in our laboratory (Pharma Serv1 (2007) and Pharma Serv 2 (2010) (unpublished data) focused on clopidogrel and SR26334 quantification; d3-clopidogrel was used as internal standard.

Table 1. Clopidogrel carboxylic acid main PK data

Author/source	Administered dose	Mean C_{max} (ng/mL)	Mean AUC_{0-t} (ng/mL*h)	Median T_{half} (h)
Lagorce (1998)	75 mg	2700.00	N/A	6.2
Hanna Ksycinska (2006)	75 mg	3200.00	8100.00	10.0
Pharma Serv 1 (2007)	75 mg	2807.81	8386.80	7.8
EMA/CHMP/595926/2010 – Study 07-197 (2007)	75 mg	2608.90	6674.70	N/A
El Ahmady et al. (2009)	75 mg	3501.00	9170.00	6.3
Pharma Serv 2 (2010)	75 mg	3164.84	10554.95	9.7
Marta Karazniewicz-Łada (2012)	75 mg	2821.00	9782.00	N/A
von Beckerath et al. (2005)	300mg	18000.00	35765.50	N/A
	adjusted to 75 mg*	4500.00	8941.38	
von Beckerath et al. (2005)	600mg	42000.00	97236.00	N/A
	adjusted to 75 mg*	5250.00	12154.50	
Yousef et al. (2013)	600 mg	24490.00	90400.00	4.3
	adjusted to 75 mg*	3061.25	11300.00	-
von Beckerath et al. (2005)	900mg	45000.00	129825.00	N/A
	adjusted to 75 mg*	3750.00	10818.75	

*Assuming dose-linearity.

Karazniewicz-Łada et al. (2012) describe a simultaneous determination of clopidogrel, SR26334 and 2 isomers of the active thiol metabolite. The clean-up of plasma samples was performed either by protein precipitation (Pharma Serv studies, Von Beckenrath et al., Lada et al.), by solid-phase extraction (Ksycinska et al.) or liquid-liquid extraction (Yousef et al.).

As it can be seen, quite similar results were obtained by different groups, irrespective of the analytical technique selected. An evaluation of PK dose linearity (see Table 2) was then carried out, based on mean of all studies for each dose strength reported in Table 1; according to the current Guideline on the Investigation of Bioequivalence (CPMP/EWP/QWP/1401/98 Rev. 1/ Corr**) assessment of dose linearity should consider whether differences in dose-adjusted AUC meet a criterion of ± 25%.

Table 2. Evaluation of dose linearity for clopidogrel carboxylic acid

Administered dose	AUC_{0-t} value adjusted to 75 mg	% mean AUC_{0-t} (AUC_{0-t} adjusted * 100/ AUC_{0-t} observed for 75 mg)	Dose linearity
300mg	8941.38	101.86	YES
600mg	11727.00	133.59	NO
900mg	10818.75	123.25	YES

A mean pharmacokinetic curve of clopidogrel carboxylic acid obtained in our lab after clopidogrel 75 mg administration in 12 healthy volunteers, in fasting conditions, is presented in Figure 2.

While it seems that from an analytical perspective, clopidogrel carboxylic acid is a desirable PK endpoint, due to the fact that reproducible results are obtained irrespective of the methodology employed, the question that still remains to be considered is whether there is any merit to this approach from a pharmacological point of view, especially keeping in mind that the metabolic pathways leading to the formation of the carboxylic acid and respectively the thiol-active metabolite are different.

Table 3 presents a similar PK comparison that has been carried out for clopidogrel itself. It is interesting to observe that an almost linear relationship between AUC_{0-t} and administered dose has been found from 75 mg and 900 mg. The situation is quite different from that of the previous table on clopidogrel carboxylic acid; PK parameters differ by a factor of 6-7 at the same administered dose (studies at different dosages were corrected for 75 mg assuming dose-PK linear response), and this fact can be seen also in two studies performed by our group. Although all authors used HPLC-MS/MS as analytical technique, plasma samples preparation was carried out either by liquid-liquid extraction (Robinson et al., Nirogi et al.) or protein precipitation at room temperature or in cold conditions (Pharma Serv studies, Taubert and Von Beckenrath group).

These PK differences between studies were already observed in the past and brought to the conclusion that in the case of clopidogrel, metabolites back-conversion in biological samples can play an important role and the measured concentrations can be highly influenced by storage, transport and processing methods.

These findings determined also the regulatory authorities to enforce particular stability and re-conversion studies in method validations for clopidogrel quantification, like mentioned in the previous section.

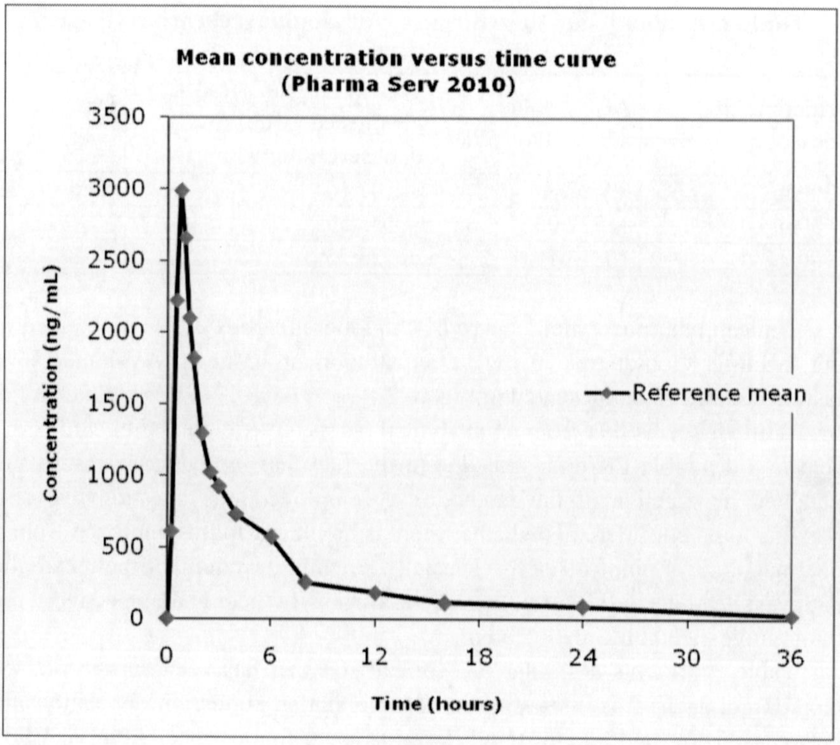

Figure 2. Mean concentration of SR26334 in 12 subjects orally treated with clopidogrel 75 mg.

Table 3. Clopidogrel main PK data

Author/Source	Administered dose	Subject selection by genotype	Mean C_{max} (ng/mL)	Mean $AUC_{0\text{-}t}$ (ng/mL*h)	Median T_{half} (h)
Nirogi (2006)	75mg (fasting)	NO	1.019	1.764	N/A
	75mg (fed)	NO	6.273	17.105	N/A
EMA/CHMP/595926/2010 - Study 07-197 (2007)	75 mg (fasting)	NO	0.9814	1.9097	N/A
Pharma Serv Study 3 (2008)	75 mg	NO	0.8032	1.8133	7.8
Pharma Serv Study 4 (2008)	75 mg	NO	1.2395	1.9175	8.5
EMA/CHMP/595926/2010 - Study 80430 (2009)	75 mg (fed-normocaloric)	NO	3.0029	5.5469	5.39

Author/Source	Administered dose	Subject selection by genotype	Mean Cmax (ng/mL)	Mean AUC0-t (ng/mL*h)	Median Thalf (h)
Pharma Serv Study 5 (2009)	75 mg (fed-high fat; high calories)	NO	4.8901	10.4251	6.8
Pharma Serv Study 6 (2009)	75 mg	NO	1.4163	2.4808	6.2
UK/H/1662/001/DC (2010)	75 mg	NO	0.9986	2.0242	N/A
Pharma Serv Study 2 (2010)	75 mg	NO	1.3990	2.6590	2.1
Robinson et al. (2007)	150 mg	NO	2.1285	4.4090	N/A
	dose adjusted to 75 mg		1.0645	2.2045	
von Beckerath et al. (2005)	300mg	NO	12.53	28.58	N/A
	dose adjusted to 75 mg (assuming dose linearity)		3.13	7.15	
Taubert et al. (2006)	300mg (dose adjusted to 75 mg (assuming dose linearity)*	3435T/T	8.6 (2.15)	11.35 (2.84)	N/A
		3435C/T and 3435C/C	14.4 (3.60)	35.58 (8.90)	
von Beckerath et al. (2005)	600mg	NO	39.25	74.40	N/A
	dose adjusted to 75 mg (assuming dose linearity)		4.91	9.30	
Taubert et al. (2006)	600mg (dose adjusted to 75 mg (assuming dose linearity)*	3435T/T	13.3 (1.66)	25.03 (3.13)	N/A
		3435C/T and 3435C/C	49.7 (6.21)	117.62 (14.70)	
von Beckerath et al. (2005)	900mg	NO	46.25	91.88	N/A
	dose adjusted to 75 mg (assuming dose linearity)		3.85	7.66	
Taubert et al. (2006)	900mg (dose adjusted to 75 mg (assuming dose linearity)*	3435T/T	55 (4.58)	142.27 (11.86)	N/A
		3435C/T and 3435C/C	34.7 (2.89)	93.03 (7.75)	

*In this work, the authors tested the hypothesis that the intestinal efflux transporter P-glycoprotein (P-gp) limits the oral bioavailability of clopidogrel and that variance in the MDR1 gene encoding P-gp predicts absorption variability. Results were presented in correlation with the MDR1 genotype subjects pertain to.

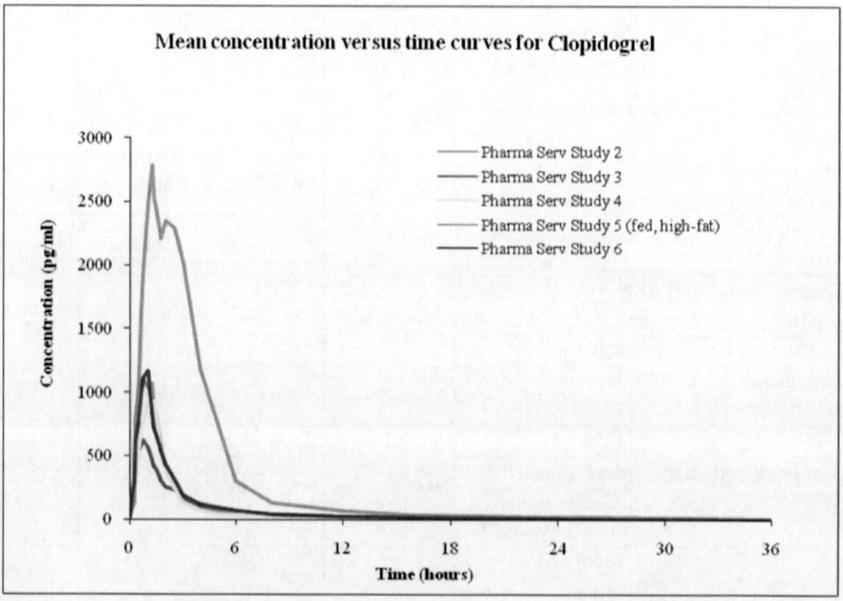

Figure 3. Mean clopidogrel concentrations obtained in 5 studies with a fixed dose of 75 mg.

Mean pharmacokinetic curves of clopidogrel obtained in the bioequivalence studies performed in our lab with a fixed dose of 75 mg per os are presented in Figure 3.

3. Clopidogrel Analytical Challenges

In 2007 our group started the development and validated an analytical method to quantify clopidogrel and clopidogrel carboxylic acid in plasma samples of subjects involved in bioequivalence studies; the classical FDA bioanalytical validation rules (2001) were followed. A fully validated method based on protein precipitation with trichloroacetic acid 20% in water/methanol 1/1 (v/v) was applied to a pharmacokinetic study. While analyzing the clinical samples, it was observed that reinjecting the extracts after an overnight stay in the autosampler, in the conditions validated with spiked plasma QCs (10°C), clopidogrel concentrations were definitively higher (more than double) than those measured in the first run. The measured concentrations of SR26334 metabolite on the other hand were stable.

Prompted by these results, a second method to determine only clopidogrel in plasma was validated, using incurred samples of real subjects in order to verify the plasma sample and extract stability. Setting of an unusually low autosampler temperature (-5ºC) was needed to obtain reproducible results in clinical samples, in contrast to the results achievable in blank plasma spiked with clopidogrel and/or SR26334 standards, which didn't show any issue. Here we must note that in this method the precipitation agent was changed to acetonitrile; still, the solution of internal standard (d3-clopidogrel) added to the samples was prepared in methanol. The problems that arose in these studies prompted us to perform, first, back-conversion tests of the metabolites described in literature (clopidogrel carboxylic acid, oxo-clopidogrel, clopidogrel active metabolite), diluted in plasma and stored or processed in different conditions. In all these experiments, clopidogrel was not measured; therefore it is evident that other metabolites from those of the known metabolic pathway could be responsible for back-conversion. In parallel, we have performed back-conversion tests on incurred samples and developed and validated a third analytical method, involving a clean-up step of the supernatant resulted from protein precipitation on HybridSPE-Precipitation 96-well plates (containing 50 mg bed). Although the internal standard solution was also prepared in methanol, the extracts were stable at 10°C, no back-conversion was observed and measured clopidogrel concentrations were reproducible, so it can be concluded that the metabolite (or metabolites) generating back-conversion were retained in the SPE-Precipitation plate (Silvestro et al., 2010).

Further studies of urine or plasma from healthy volunteers treated with a high oral dosage of clopidogrel (8 x 75 mg) revealed a series of other metabolites scarcely described in the literature. Among them, clopidogrel acyl glucuronide, initially identified from the mass spectrum, and subsequently confirmed with a commercially available standard, was recognized as the major source of back-conversion (Silvestro et al., 2011). The results of clopidogrel acyl glucuronide stability tests in different solvents (all dilutions at a concentration of 1μg/mL), pH and temperatures showed a very high rate of back-conversion, probably through transmethylation, in alkaline conditions in methanol (resulting clopidogrel concentrations up to 300ng/ml); acidic conditions were also favoring the back-conversion. Even at neutral pH the measured clopidogrel concentration was 11 ng/mL after 24 h at room temperature; at lower temperature (4 ºC) the back-conversion rate decreased with 85% (1.5 ng/mL).

This behavior of the acyl glucuronide metabolite is in agreement with the results described in a few papers (Yerino et al. (2006), Garofolo et al. (2009)).

The transesterification between the glucuronide group and the methanol used in sample preparation (to dilute the internal standard and/or for protein precipitation) was the cause of these unexpected results and in fact a method avoiding the use of methanol during sample preparation and chromatographic separation showed optimal validation results; a schema of the chemical reactions involved in this back-conversion process is presented in Figure 4.

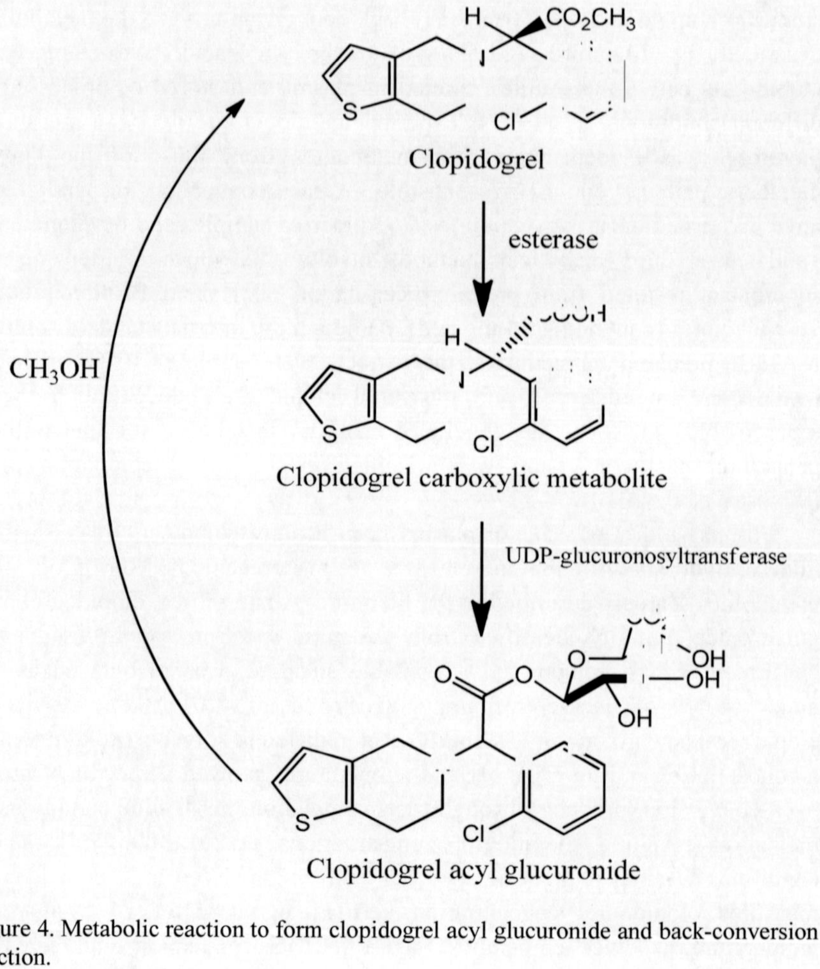

Figure 4. Metabolic reaction to form clopidogrel acyl glucuronide and back-conversion reaction.

As it can be expected, ethanol or isopropanol also produce transesterification; however the reaction products differ from clopidogrel. It is notewhorty that the reactivity decreases significantly (10 to 100 fold) with the increase of the alkyl chain length [Silvestro et al. (2011)].

In any case methanol should be avoided when analysing clopidogrel in biological fluids, keeping in mind that the concentrations of clopidogrel acyl-glucuronide in those fluids are about 500-fold higher than the concentrations of clopidogrel itself (details in the next section).

4. Experimental Data on Clopidogrel Acyl Glucuronide PK

Clarified that clopidogrel acyl glucuronide metabolite plays a critical role in the analytical back-conversion problems observed in clopidogrel quantification, it was interesting to evaluate its PK profile in plasma and compare it with clopidogrel and clopidogrel carboxylic acid PK.

We have then established a new method for the simultaneous quantification of all three analytes (clopidogrel acyl-glucuronide, clopidogrel carboxylic acid and clopidogrel) in plasma using the best conditions to avoid back-conversion; clopidogrel-d_3 was added as internal standard (Silvestro et al. (2011)).

Later, the method was revalidated and a second internal standard, clopidogrel carboxylic acid-$^{13}C_6$, was introduced beside d3-clopidogrel, in order to compensate properly the matrix effects for the two metabolites, eluting very early compared to clopidogrel retention time. A representative chromatogram is presented in Figure 5.

Samples from 10 subjects included in a bioequivalence study with clopidogrel 75mg, administered orally and in single dose, were analysed with this method. PK data (semilogarithmic plot) for clopidogrel acyl-glucuronide are presented in Figure 6 in comparison to the data obtained in the same study for clopidogrel and clopidogrel carboxylic acid; mean PK variables are available in Table 5.

It is interesting to observe that the exposure to this metabolite in man, based on $AUC_{0\text{-}inf}$ data, is practically 500 times higher than that observed in the same subjects for clopidogrel and 6 times lower than that of clopidogrel carboxylic acid.

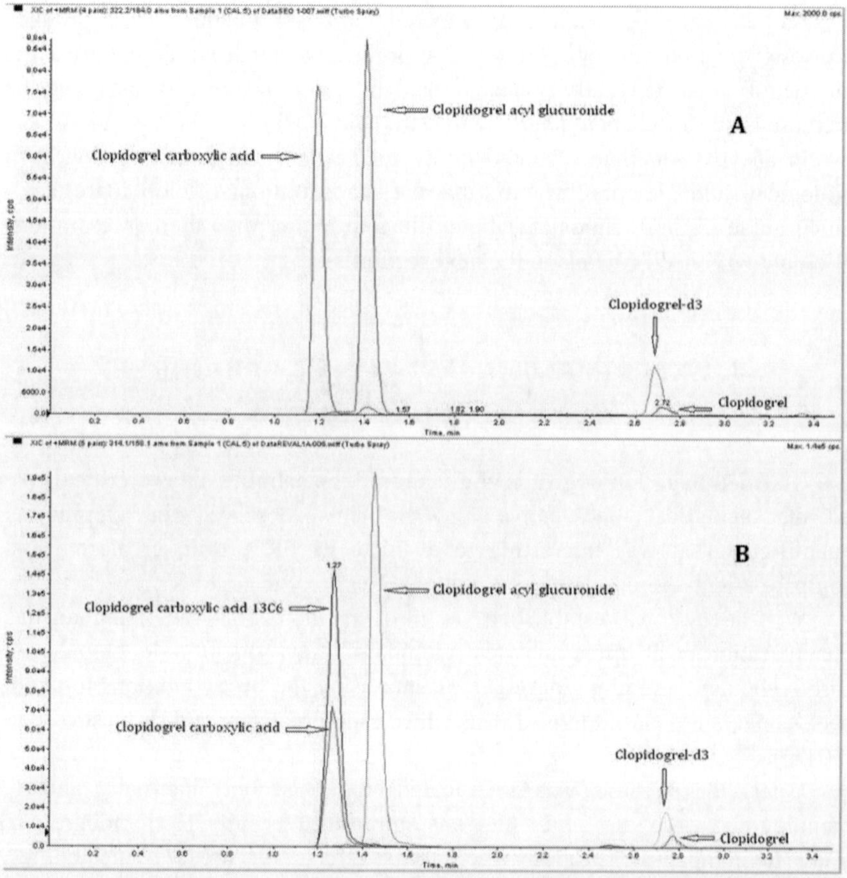

Figure 5. (A) Chromatograms recorded on the MRM transitions of clopidogrel (322.2/184.0), clopidogrel-d3 (327.2/189.2), clopidogrel carboxylic acid (308.2/95.0), and clopidogrel acyl glucuronide (484.3/198.1) after the injection of a spiked sample precipitated with acetonitrile. (B) Chromatograms of the same method, revalidated adding clopidogrel carboxylic acid $^{13}C_6$ (314.1/158.1) as internal standard for the early-eluting analytes. Mass spectrometer: AB Sciex API 4000Qtrap. Column: Ascentis Express RP-Amide (100x2.1 mm, 5μm). Mobile phase: gradient of formic acid 0.1% in water and acetonitrile, at a flow rate of 0.2 mL/min. Injection volume: 10μL.

Little other information is available on clopidogrel acyl glucuronide. A poster by Yerino et al. showed in 2006 that this metabolite has a modest activity as CYP2C8 inhibitor, while a very recent work [Inoue et al. (2013)] evaluating the inhibitory effect of this acyl glucuronide metabolite on human carboxylesterases concluded that it selectively inhibits hCES1 but not hCES2.

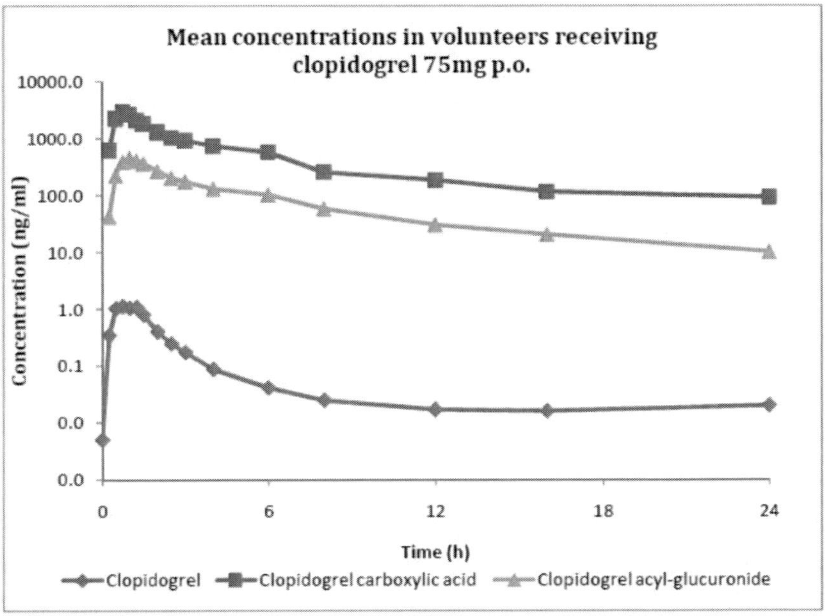

Figure 6. PK curve of clopidogrel acyl-glucuronide, SR26334 and clopidogrel.

Besides this, no other data is available and, in particular, it is unclear if this metabolite is mainly excreted in urine, bile or both elimination pathways. It is interesting to remember that, in case of a biliary excretion, an entero-hepatic circulation can be expected, bringing to a prolonged half-life of the carboxylic acid metabolite in plasma.

5. Clopidogrel Active Metabolite PK

Pioneering work on clopidogrel active metabolite PK was presented by the group of Taubert and Von Beckenrath in 2004 and 2005. They have used high loading dose of medication (300, 600 and 900 mg) and a tentative quantification of the active metabolite was achieved employing a surrogate calibration curve of clopidogrel (an appropriate standard was not commercially available).

Analyses were carried out with LC-MS/MS, the sample preparation was performed by protein precipitation, and 1-methyl-4-phenylpyridinium bromide was added as internal standand.

As it can be seen in Table 4, that resumes the data available so far on clopidogrel active metabolite PK, the plasma concentrations were very low in these first studies, probably due to the thiol metabolite instability but more likely to the already mentioned analytical drawbacks of using a surrogate calibration curve and non-labeled internal standard.

Takahasi et al. described in 2008 the first validated method using an active metabolite analytical standard. They also applied LC-MS/MS and, in order to stabilize the thiol group, a derivatization reaction with 2-bromo-3-methoxy-acetophenone was carried out just after blood sample collection. A 4-bromo-acetophenone analog of clopidogrel active metabolite was added as internal standard prior to the solid-phase extraction clean-up. It is important to observe that the derivatization approach was partially pushed by the consideration that the active metabolite containing a thiol is a highly reactive compound with critical aspects of stability. Interestingly, the group of Taubert, in a German patent application to cover a specific method of samples stabilization, showed that in adequate cold conditions the active metabolite has an acceptable stability in plasma, while it is definitively unstable at ambient temperature [DE 10 2004 046 159 A1 (2006)]. Later in 2010 three groups (Delavenne et al., Furlong et al., Lada et al.) have published new studies on clopidogrel active metabolite PK. All authors followed the same approach of Takahasi and used 2-bromo-3-methoxy-acetophenone to stabilize the thiol in blood samples. It is important to mention that 4 isomers of this active metabolite were already observed in the first study "in vitro" of Savi et al. in 2000 and only one was active; the groups of Lada et al. and Furlong et al. dedicated particular attention to this fact, thus observing that in plasma samples only form 3 and 4 were present (only form 4 is active). A quantification method developed and fully validated (unpublished data) in our laboratory in about the same period was based on a similar analytical approach, but without derivatization and with sample handling at very low temperatures. Plasma storage was at -70°C and processing (by simple protein precipitation with acetonitrile) at 2-4°C. Samples were analyzed by HPLC-MS/MS following the fragmentation of the protonated ions from clopidogrel active metabolite (MRM transition 356.1/212.2) and its deuterated analogue (d_3) used as internal standard; in the case of the later, the isotope ^{37}Cl was used (MRM transition 361.1/217.1). Both the active metabolite used for the calibration curves and quality controls, and the internal standard were obtained *in vitro* as described by Savi et al. (2000) starting from synthetic oxo-clopidogrel (d_3-oxo-clopidogrel in case of the internal standard), purified and quantified by inductive coupled plasma-

MS; the method selectively measured only the active form (4) of this metabolite.

Representative chromatograms are presented in Figure 7.

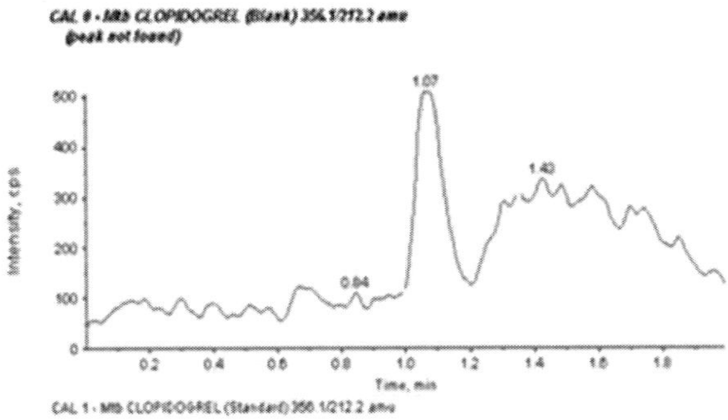

a

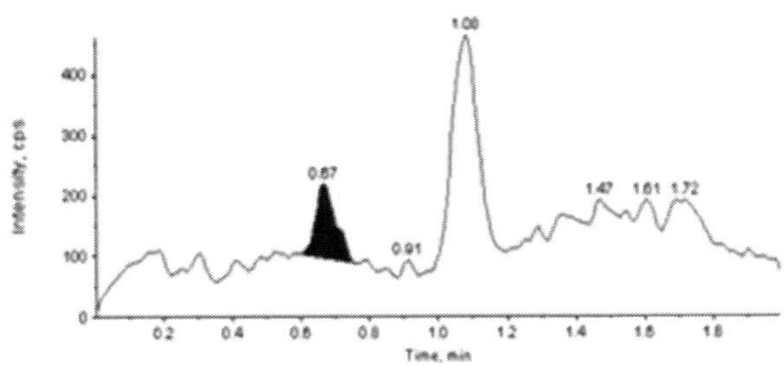

b

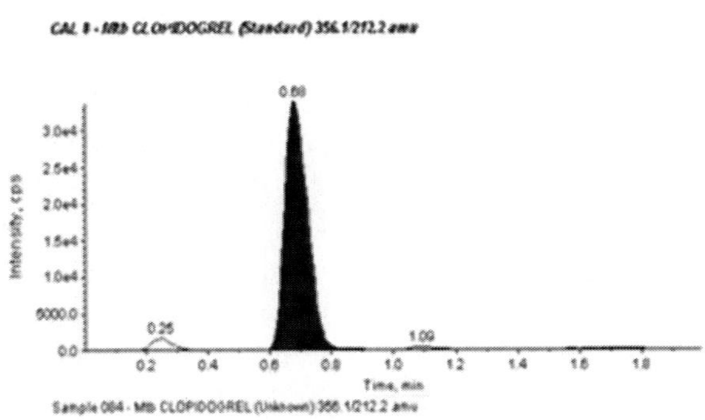

c

Figure 7. (Continued)

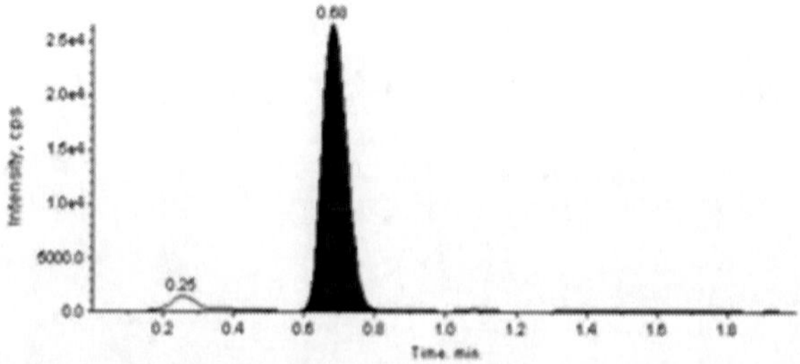

d

Figure 7. Chromatograms of clopidogrel active metabolite in blank plasma (A), plasma spiked at Cal 1 - 100 pg/mL (B), Cal 8- 60000 pg/mL (C) and in a sample from a subject treated with clopidogrel 75 mg (D). Mass spectrometer: AB Sciex API 5000. Column: Ascentis Express RP-Amide (100x2.1 mm, 5µm) maintained at 35°C. Mobile phase: gradient of (A) formic acid 0.1% in water/methanol 65/35 (v/v) and (B), formic acid 0.1% in water/methanol 10/90(v/v) at a flow rate of 0.25 mL/min. Injection volume: 20µL.

To help understanding the first results of Taubert et al., Figure 8 presents plasma concentrations obtained in one of our PK studies (clopidogrel dose 75 mg, fasting conditions), as first determined in 2008 using a surrogate calibration curve of clopidogrel (according to the method described by Taubert in 2004) and as determined again in 2009, using a calibration curve of clopidogrel active metabolite. As it can be observed, a substantial underestimation of active metabolite concentration occurs when using a surrogate calibration curve. It is interesting to note that results obtained in our laboratory in 2009 are in good agreement with those obtained by the authors using derivatization while the original results from 2008 closely resemble those of Taubert et al. and von Beckerath et al. (see Table 4).

Among the presented studies, the one performed by von Beckerath (2005) took into consideration the aspect of PK linearity for the active metabolite, within the dose range of 300 to 900mg clopidogrel, following the administration of a single loading dose. Due to the fact that only three distinct doses were administered, no clear statistical evaluation of linearity can be made. However, it seems easily noticeable that from 300 to 600 mg the PK is almost linear, while the dose increase from 600 to 900mg (150%) results in only modest increase in C_{max} (108.4%) and $AUC_{0\text{-}t}$ (137.8%), suggesting a saturation of the metabolism.

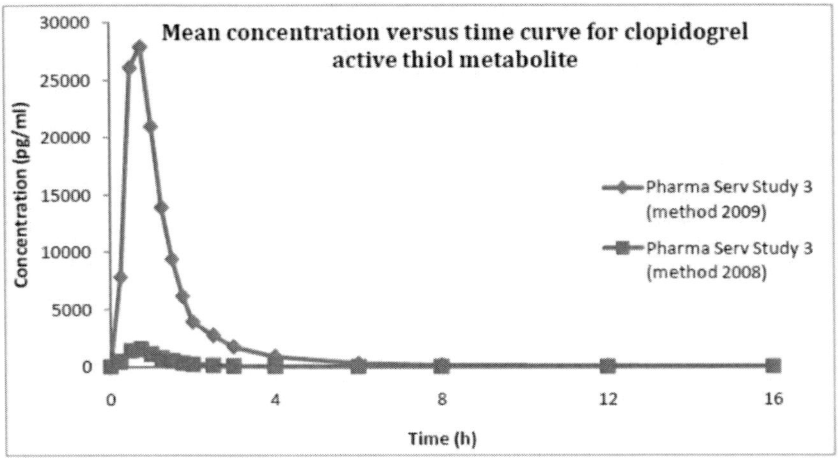

Figure 8. PK curve of clopidogrel active metabolite, same study (single dose, 75mg), quantified using two distinct analytical methods.

Table 4. Clopidogrel active thiol metabolite main PK data

Author/source	Administered dose	Subject selection by genotype	Mean C_{max} (ng/mL)	Mean AUC_{0-t} (ng/mL*h)	Median T_{half} (h)
Pharma Serv Study 3 (2008)	75 mg	NO	(2008[1]): 1.669	(2008[1]): 1.815	(2008[1]): 0.65
			(2009[2]): 30.915	(2009[2]): 35.383	(2009[2]): 1.14
Pharma Serv Study 5 (2009)	75 mg (fed)	NO	19.6240	34.6131	1.48
Karazniewicz-Łada et al. (2012)	75 mg	NO	H3 isomer: 14.8	H3 isomer: 18.6	0.58
			H4 isomer: 13.3	H4 isomer: 16.6	0.57
			Total: 28.1	Total: 35.2	
Furlog et al. (2013)	75 mg***	NO	H4 isomer 11.0	H4 isomer AUC_{0-12}: 11.5	0.97
von Beckerath et al. (2005)	300mg	NO	2.82	4.35	N/A
	adjusted to 75mg (assuming dose linearity)		0.71	1.09	
Taubert et al. (2006)	300mg	3435T/T carriers	1.20	1.88	N/A

Table 4. (Continued)

Author/source	Administered dose	Subject selection by genotype	Mean C_{max} (ng/mL)	Mean AUC_{0-t} (ng/mL*h)	Median T_{half} (h)
Taubert et al. (2006)	300mg	3435C/T and 3435C/C	3.20	7.85	N/A
Takahashi et al. (2008)	300mg	NO	35.9	43.8 (AUC_{0-inf})*	0.52
	adjusted to 75mg (assuming dose linearity)		8.975	10.95	N/A
von Beckerath et al. (2005)	600mg	NO	5.85	8.30	N/A
	adjusted to 75 mg (assuming dose linearity)		0.73	1.04	
Taubert et al. (2006)	600mg	3435T/T carriers	2.50	3.48	N/A
		3435C/T and 3435C/C	6.60	12.40	N/A
Delavenne et al. (2010)	600mg	NO	82.60	131.5 (AUC_{0-inf})*	0.4
	adjusted to 75mg (assuming dose linearity)		10.33	16.44	
von Beckerath et al. (2005)	900mg	NO	6.34	11.43	N/A
	adjusted to 75mg (assuming dose linearity)		0.53	0.95	
Taubert et al. (2006)	900mg	3435T/T carriers	7.30	16.90	N/A
		3435C/T and 3435C/C	5.40	10.55	N/A

*Considering the short half-life of the active metabolite and the fact that the sampling schedule was long, basically the value listed can be considered AUC0-t since no extrapolation is needed in the given study conditions.

**In this work, the authors tested the hypothesis that the intestinal efflux transporter P-glycoprotein (P-gp) limits the oral bioavailability of clopidogrel and that variance in the MDR1 gene encoding P-gp predicts absorption variability. Results are presented in correlation with the MDR1 genotype subjects pertain to.

***Treatment schedule: 600 mg clopidogrel loading dose on day 1, followed by once daily dosing of 75 mg on days 2 through 5. Pk samples collected on Day 5.

6. Experimental Data on Oxo-Clopidogrel PK

Despite the fact that this metabolite has been for a long time known as a key intermediate in the formation of the clopidogrel active metabolite, PK data on 2-oxo-clopidogrel are, according to our knowledge, unavailable so far. In 2013 we have developed and partially validated a HPLC-MS/MS analytical method for its determination in plasma. 2-oxo-clopidogrel and the internal standard, 2-oxo-clopidogrel-d3, were monitored on the MRM transitions 338.1/155.1 and 341.1/158.0, respectively. Sample clean-up was carried out by acetonitrile protein precipitation, in cold conditions; representative chromatograms are presented in figure 9. Preliminary experiments on 2-oxo-clopidogrel stability didn't show special problems in neat standard solutions, but degradation occured in biological samples; the optimal conditions for long term plasma storage and sample processing are still under evaluation.

Samples from a PK study with administration of 75 mg clopidogrel have been analyzed shortly after collection, in order to minimize degradation problems; the PK results are resumed in Figure 10 and PK data values are summarized in Table 5.

As it can be seen, the levels are quite similar to those obtained for the active metabolite (as presented in the same figure). We don't have at the moment any correlation to PD data or PK linearity information. In any case, this preliminary work has shown the feasibility of this determination and opens the direction for future interesting experiments of PK/PD correlations as well as the possibility to evaluate directly if the limiting metabolic rate step is from clopidogrel to 2-oxo-clopidogrel, from 2-oxo-clopidogrel to the active metabolite, or both are critical.

7. Considerations on Other Potential Metabolites of Clopidogrel

Other oxidative metabolites can be expected, in particular hydroxyl derivatives of clopidogrel. At the moment no data has been published showing the presence of such metabolites; these compounds can be also a starting point for additional conjugate metabolites.

Interestingly, the active thiol metabolite of clopidogrel can also participate to the formation of thiol derivatives (with glutathione, cysteine etc.) whose existence is yet unclear.

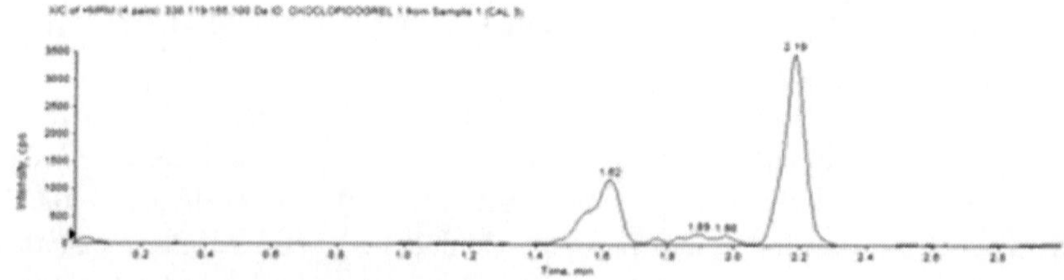

a

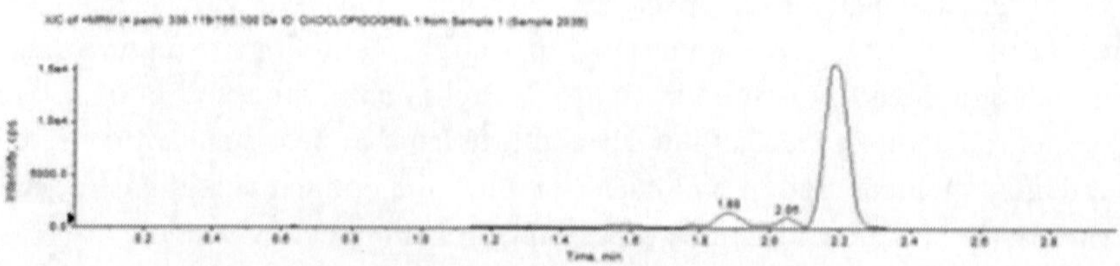

b

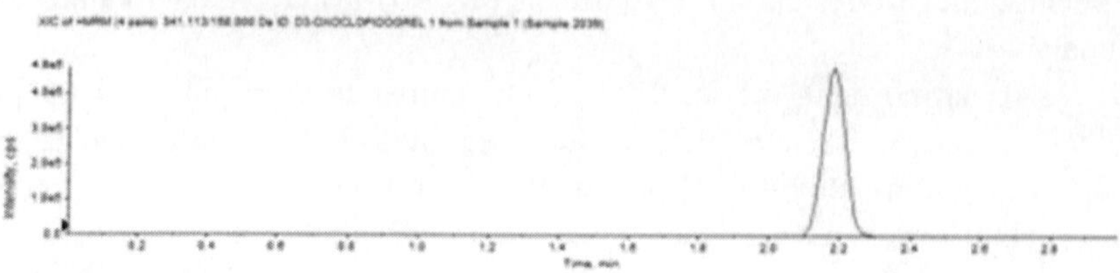

c

Figure 9. Chromatograms recorded on the MRM transitions of 2-oxo-clopidogrel (338.1/155.1) and 2-oxo-clopidogrel-d3 (341.1/158.0) after the injection of a spiked sample (A) and an incurred sample (B) precipitated with acetonitrile. The peak of the internal standard in the incurred sample is shown panel (C). Mass spectrometer: API 4000 Qtrap. Column: Ascentis Express RP-Amide (100x2.1 mm, 5µm) maintained at 55°C. Mobile phase: gradient of formic acid 0.1% in water and acetonitrile at a flow rate of 0.2 mL/min. Injection volume: 10µL.

A few experiments performed in our laboratory to measure the active clopidogrel metabolite after reduction of plasma samples with dithiotreitol to release the conjugates showed levels 30 to 50% higher than the ones obtained without reduction.

These few data seems to prove the existence of such conjugates; an additional aspect to be studied is also the binding to sulfhidryl compounds present in cells and tissue. All together, the clopidogrel metabolism can still offer interesting areas of investigation.

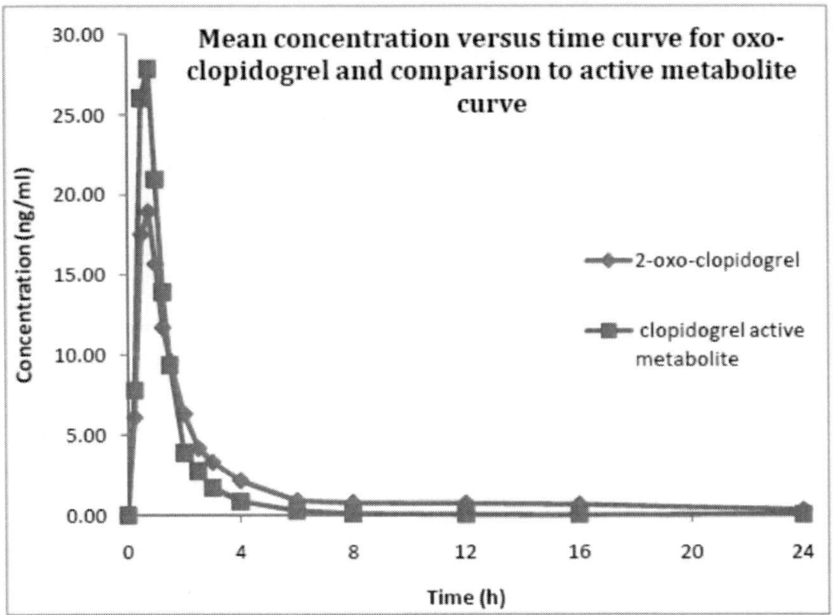

Figure 10. Pharmacokinetic curve of 2-oxo-clopidogrel (samples collected from 5 volunteers treated with clopidogrel 75 mg).

8. Overall Vision of Clopidogrel Metabolism and PK

The conversion of clopidogrel to its active metabolite is mediated by multiple P450 cytochromes, as aforementioned in the beginning of this chapter. There are 3 major CYP2C19 genetic polymorphisms. CYP2C19*1 corresponds to normal function. CYP2C19*2 and CYP2C19*3 are loss-of-function alleles and explain most of the reduced function in subjects who are poor metabolizers. CYP2C19*2 and *3 account for 85% and 99% of the nonfunctional alleles in whites and Asians, respectively. Poor metabolizers have 2 loss-of-function alleles. Intermediate metabolizers have 1 copy of a loss-of-function allele and may also have decreased active metabolite levels and reduced anti-platelet aggregation effects when treated with clopidogrel, but FDA's boxed warning only refers to poor metabolizers (Holmes et al. (2010)). It should however be noted that although the warning emphasizes the fact that there is indeed a higher risk associated with the use of clopidogrel in poor metabolizers, it does not specifically require genetic testing nor does it state that the drug should be contraindicated in such patients. A plausible reason would be that so far it has been shown that the relation between CYP2C19*2 genotype and platelet aggregation merely accounts for 12% of the overall variation in the response to clopidogrel therapy (Shuldiner et al. (2009)).

Another potential source of variability was recently proposed by Bouman et al. (2011) who identified paraoxonase-1 (PON1) as a major determinant of the bioconversion of clopidogrel with its common Q192R polymorphism determining the rate of active thiol metabolite formation. The paper concluded that PON1 Q192R polymorphism explained 72.5% of the variability in ADP-stimulated platelet aggregation after clopidogrel administration. However, after having genotyped PON1 (Q192R and L55M) and CYP2C19 variants in 106 patients enrolled in the PK/PD CLOVIS-2 trial, Hulot et al. (2011) have concluded that the results do not support an important contribution of PON1 Q192R and L55M as major determinants of clopidogrel PK and PD responsiveness. Nevertheless, because CYP2C19 seems to explain only a minor part of clopidogrel bioactivation, future studies to unravel the pharmacogenetics of clopidogrel are highly warranted [Jaapjan (2011)].

Furthermore, another recently proposed key contributor to the inter-individual variability in response to clopidogrel is hepatic carboxylesterase 1 (CES1) whose single nucleotide polymorphisms (SNPs) G143E (rs71647871) and D260fs (rs71647872) have been shown to exhibit markedly decreased enzymatic activity towards the hydrolysis of some CES1 substrates (eg. methylphenidate, oseltamivir, trandolapril) [Zhu et al. (2012)]. It was therefore hypothesised that clopidogrel metabolism may also be affected by variability in the expresion of the enzyme, given that hydrolysis of clopidogrel prodrug to the inactive metabolite clopidogrel carboxylic acid is catalized by CES1 and this reaction accounts for the fate of 85% of an administered dose of clopidogrel. Subsequently the ~15% of a clopidogrel dose that remains available undergoes further oxidative metabolism catalyzed by cytochrome P450 (CYP) 1A2, 2B6, and 2C19, with formation of 2-oxo-clopidogrel which is again subject to concurring reactions; a part of it is hydrolyzed by CES1 to form 2-oxo-clopidogrel carboxylate, an inactive metabolite, and the balance of 2-oxo-clopidogrel is further hydrolyzed to the unstable but active 5-thiol metabolite. Hao-Jie Zhu et al. wanted to determine whether CES1 inhibition and *CES1* genetic polymorphisms would significantly influence the biotransformation of clopidogrel and alter formation of the active metabolite, as could be asumed when considering its involvment in the biotransformation of clopidogrel. Their conclusion was that deficient CES1 catalytic activity resulting from CES1 inhibition or *CES1* genetic variation may be associated with higher plasma concentrations of clopidogrel active metabolite and hence, enhanced antiplatelet activity.

Following upon the research of Kuzui et al. (2010) and more to the point, on the obervation that in-vitro formation of the active metabolite of clopidogrel from 2-oxo-clopidogrel required the addition of reduced glutathione (GSH) as substrate, Zhang et al. tried to establish whether a correlation can be found between varying glutathione concentrations and the amount of thiol metabolite formed. Based on the group's previous work, where the formation of a glutathionyl conjugate of the active metabolite of clopidogrel was reported, it was established that a relevant correlation would have to account for both the active metabolite formation as well as its glutathionyl conjugate. It has already been established that clopidogrel is bioactivated through two sequential oxidative processes, the first one resulting in the formation of 2-2-oxo-clopidogrel which has no antiplatelet activity. Subsequently, in the second step, 2-oxo clopidogrel is further oxidized to give an unstable sulfenic acid intermediate. Reduction of the sulfenic acid by GSH leads to thiolactone ring opening to form a glutathionyl conjugate followed by a thiol-disulfide exchange to form the thiol active metabolite. It is currently unknown whether the glutathionyl conjugate of clopidogrel exhibits antiplatelet activity, but the results of the study do indicate that the formation of both the active metabolite and the glutathionyl conjugate exhibit similar saturation kinetics, indicating that formation of the glutathionyl conjugate constitutes an integral part of the bioactivation processes of 2-oxo clopidogrel via CYP-catalyzed reactions [Zhang et al. (2012)].

It is therefore suggested that the levels of active metabolite may be prone to changes due to factors other than P450-catalyzed reactions, such as the concentrations of GSH or other reduction agents that may be associated with oxidative stress, inflammation etc., thus potentially affecting the effective concentration of active metabolite also in vivo.

Since the premises for a discussion on potential step-limiting reactions involved in the biotransformation of clopidogrel to its active metabolite have been laid out, it is important also to do a review of the information provided by food effect studies.

In Figure 11, pharmacokinetic curves obtained for clopidogrel and the active metabolite, following the administration of a single 75mg dose in fasting and fed conditions (after intake of a high fat, high calories breakfast) are shown.

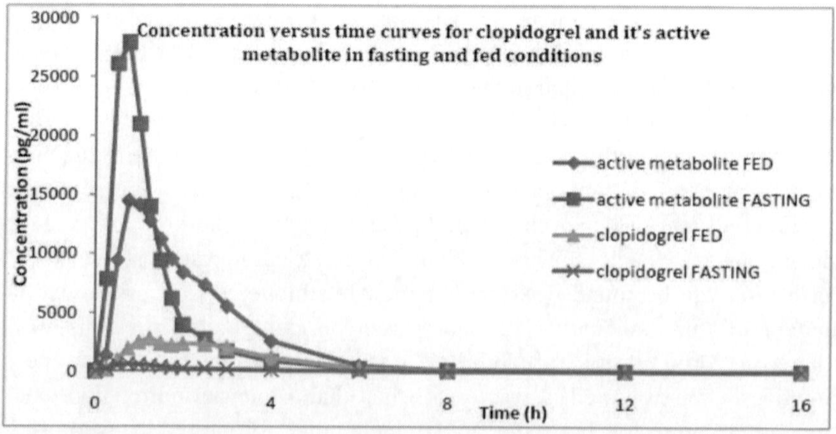

Figure 11. Concentration versus time curves for clopidogrel and its active metabolite in fasting and fed conditions.

For clopidogrel itself a significant increase is apparent with regard to both peak exposure (the ratio $C_{max\ FED}/C_{max\ FASTING}$ is 6.08) and extent (the ratio $AUC_{0\text{-}t\ FED}$ to $AUC_{0\text{-}t\ FASTING}$ is 5.75) of absorption in fed conditions, as already reported by Nirogi et al. in 2006.

For clopidogrel active metabolite, while administration in fasting conditions resulted in a peak exposure 60% higher than in fed conditions, the extent of exposure was almost identical (the ratio $AUC_{0\text{-}t\ FASTING}$ to $AUC_{0\text{-}t\ FED}$ is 1.022); in any case it is noteworthy that the increase of peak exposure and extent of exposure observed for clopidogrel didn't appear. The fact that food intake does not have a significant effect on total exposure of the active metabolite is in agreement with the pharmacodynamic findings that prompted the label claim stating that clopidogrel's effectiveness is not affected by food intake.

In conclusion, an overall summary of the proposed metabolic pathway for clopidogrel is shown in Figure 12. As it can be seen, new pathways have appeared (here represented in red color) compared to previous information available in 1998, at the time when clopidogrel was approved in the European Union. The following figures (13 and 14) and Table 5 resume the exposure parameters calculated for each metabolite (AUC and C_{max}) and the parent compound in a group of subjects receiving a standard clopidogrel dose (75 mg).

From these data it can be noticed that clopidogrel itself shows the lowest exposure, while the two oxidative metabolites, 2-oxo-clopidogrel and the active metabolite, show 25-fold and respectively 38-fold higher values with respect to peak exposure and 26-fold and respectively 20-fold higher values for extent of exposure as compared to clopidogrel.

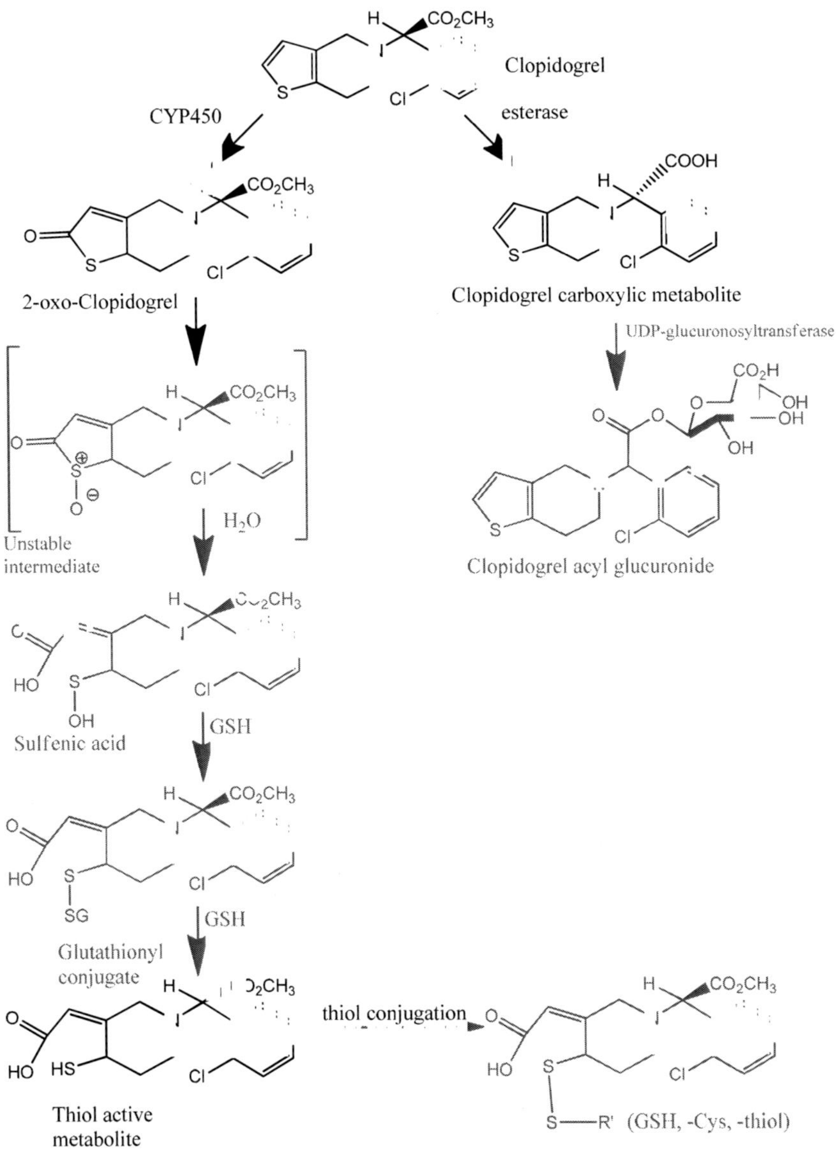

Figure 12. Clopidogrel metabolic pathway.

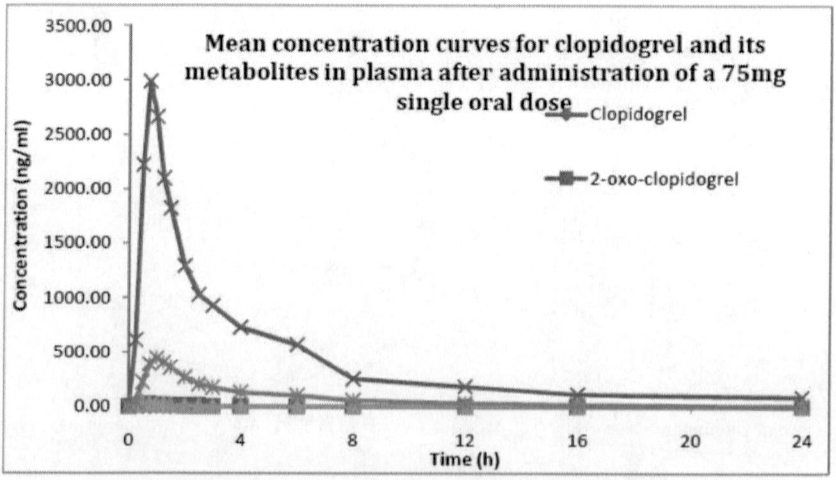

Figure 13. Linear presentation of mean PK curves for clopidogrel and metabolites.

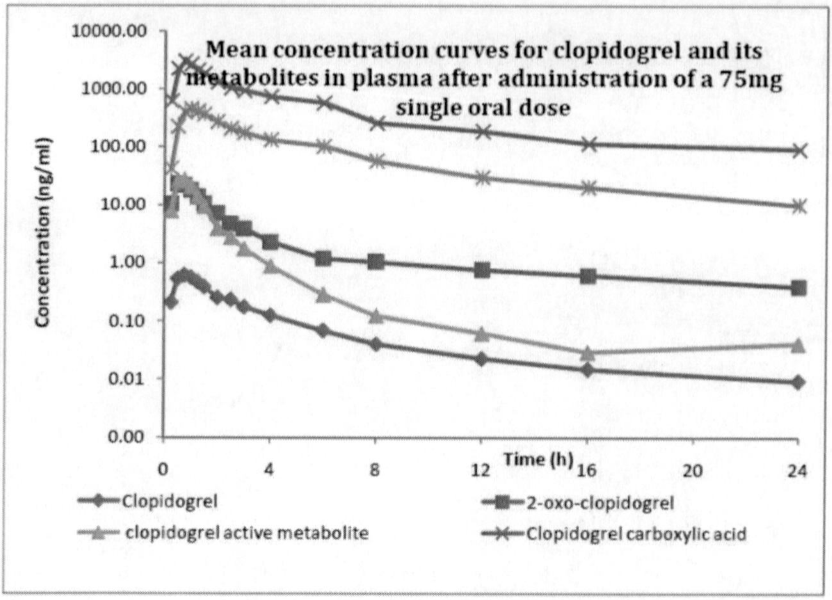

Figure 14. Semi-logarithmic presentation of mean PK curves for clopidogrel and metabolites.

Table 5. Mean PK parameters for clopidogrel and its metabolites after administration of a single 75mg oral dose in fasting conditions

Substance	Mean C_{max} (ng/ml)	Mean AUC_{0-t} (ng/ml *h)	Median T_{max} (h)	Median T_{half}
Clopidogrel (2008)	0.803	1.813	0.750	7.828
Clopidogrel active metabolite (2009)	30.915	35.383	0.750	1.143
Clopidogrel carboxylic acid (2010)	3164.835	10554.947	0.75	9.704
Clopidogrel acyl glucuronide (2010)	471.428	1706.764	1.000	6.845
2-Oxo-clopidogrel (2012)	20.390	47.353	0.750	1.800

The exposure of clopidogrel carboxylic acid and clopidogrel acyl glucuronide is definitely more significant, with C_{max} values 3940 and respectively 586 times higher than those of the prodrug and AUC_{0-t} values 5821 and respectively 941 times higher than those registered for clopidogrel itself. These data show that obviously the desesterification is a much faster and extensive metabolic reaction in comparison to the oxidative one.

9. Possible PD Impact of Clopidogrel PK

According to EMA's Q and A Paper of the Pharmacokinetics Working Party (EMA/618604/2008 Rev. 7), citing the work of Nirogi et al. (2006) as well as other unspecified studies reviewed, there are indications that in the fed state the bioavailability of a single oral dose of clopidogrel increases dramatically (500 - 600 %) while the systemic exposure to the major but inactive carboxylic acid metabolite increases only by approximately 10-20 %. The EWP-PK subgroup reviewed the solubility properties of clopidogrel salts and these indicate that when administration of clopidogrel occurs under fasting conditions, the dissolution in the gastric media with a subsequent hydrolysis and formation of the inactive carboxy-acid metabolite is maximal. As a consequence, the extent of unchanged drug that still is available for absorption (at the intestine level) is reduced. Conversely, the dissolution of clopidogrel is limited in the gastric media under fed conditions, the acidic hydrolysis in the stomach is reduced and the bioavailability of clopidogrel is improved (EMA/ 618604/2008).

As evidence would suggest, hepatic hydrolysis is saturable for clopidogrel while absorption from dosage form is not a limiting factor. Naturally, from a pharmacodynamic perspective, more important is the fate of the amount of circulating unchanged prodrug that remains available for oxidation to 2-oxo-clopidogrel and subsequent conversion to the thiol active metabolite. Based on the observations made by our group on yet unpublished data from fasting and fed bioequivalence studies on clopidogrel as well as on data published by Hurbin et. al (2012), it was concluded that, although exposure to clopidogrel increases dramatically in the fed state, extent of exposure (AUC) to the active thiol metabolite varies insignificantly. This important PK finding correlates well with the fact that clopidogrel active metabolite formation exhibits a plateau behavior (as apparent in the work of von Beckerath et al. 2005) that results also in a pharmacodynamic dose ceiling effect, as tripling the dosing from a regular loading dose of 300 mg to 900 mg produces only 60% inhibition of ADP induced platelet aggregation (Patent application EP 2540729 A1).

In conclusion, highly increased exposure to clopidogrel, either be it by increased bioavailability due to administration in fed state or by overdosing, does not result in significantly higher rate of metabolite formation, nor does it linearly correlate with increased effectiveness. Could the discrepancies between the levels of prodrug available and the thiol metabolite formed be explained by the fact that the first oxidative step involved in the metabolism of clopidogrel is saturable? Studies to provide evidence of that effect would be welcomed in the future and it might also be interesting to follow-up on the clinical developments in the case of 2-oxo-clopidogrel, which has been proposed as an anti-thrombotic medication itself in a recent patent application (EP 2540729 A1).

A work of Bouman et al. in 2009 is one of the best investigations on the PK/PD interaction for clopidogrel. In this paper, aimed in reality to evaluate the appropriateness of different platelet aggregation assessment methods, the authors have correlated the PK of clopidogrel active metabolite with a series of these tests and found a good correlation for some of them.

It is so far clear that PK data of the active metabolite can be a good predictor of therapeutic activity, but more work is needed to identify an adequate threshold for plasma concentrations that could serve for therapeutic drug monitoring. Despite the wider availability of mass spectrometers in clinical chemistry laboratories in the last years, the determination of clopidogrel active metabolite remains quite complex, especially due to the problems of sample stability, limiting its application.

Conclusion

As shown in the previous paragraphs a lot of progress has been done in the clarification of clopidogrel PK and metabolism; the situation is now adequate to perform in each subject a suitable therapeutic drug monitoring that should be most probably focused on the active metabolite. It seems interesting to evaluate this approach of therapeutic optimization, beside genotyping, due to the fact that patients often receive clopidogrel as part of complex therapies with several drugs, each influencing differently the metabolism of clopidogrel. In these conditions it is not always possible to replace all treatments with molecules without metabolic interactions and the genotype on the other side can only predict a risk, without assessing the real impact of such complex metabolic interactions.

Beside this aspect of individualized therapy, it is clear that high-tech analytical capabilities will be of help in the development of new clopidogrel derivatives and also in the optimized use of new drug combinations.

References

Bouman, H. J., Schomig, E., et al., Paraoxonase-1 is a major determinant of clopidogrel efficacy. *Nat. Med.* 17 (2011) 110–116

Bundesrepublik Deutschland Deutsches Patent- und Markenamt, Document Reference: DE 10 2004 046 159 A1; 2006.04.06

Delavenne, X., Basset, T., et al., Ultra-performance LC MS/MS method for quantification of clopidogrel active metabolite, *J. Sep. Sci.* (2010) 33: 1968–1972

El Ahmady, O., Ibrahim, M., et al., Bioequivalence of two oral formulations of clopidogrel tablets in healthy male volunteers, *Int. J. Clin. Pharmacol. Ther.* (2009) 47(12): 780-4

Furlong, M. T., Savant, I., et al., A validated HPLC-MS/MS assay for quantifying unstable pharmacologically active metabolites of clopidogrel in human plasma: Application to a clinical pharmacokinetic study, *J. Chromatogr. B Analyt. Technol. Biomed. Life Sci.* (2013) 926:36-41

Garofolo, F. (2009) Impact of unstable metabolites during drug quantification and specific evaluation of acyl glucuronide metabolites in bioanalysis. *Lecture, AAPS Symposium*, Nov. 2009

Holmes, D., et al., A Report of the American College of Cardiology Foundation Task Force on Clinical Expert Consensus Documents and the American Heart Association Endorsed by the Society for Cardiovascular Angiography and Interventions and the Society of Thoracic Surgeons, *J. Am. Coll. Cardiol.* (2010) 56(4):321-341

Hulot, J. S., Collet, J. P., CYP2C19 But Not PON1 Genetic Variants Influence Clopidogrel Pharmacokinetics, Pharmacodynamics, and Clinical Efficacy in Post–Myocardial Infarction Patients, *Circulation: Cardiovascular Interventions* (2011) 4 :422-428

Hurbin, F., Boulenc, X., et al., Clopidogrel pharmacodynamics and pharmacokinetics in the fed and fasted state: a randomized crossover study of healthy men., *J. Clin. Pharmacol.* (2012) 52(10): 1506-15

Inoue, N. R., Hall, A., et al., Reversible inhibition of human carboxylesterases by acyl glucuronides, *Drug Metab. Dispos.* (2013) 41(4): 698-703

Jaapjan, D., Unraveling the Pharmacogenetics of Clopidogrel - The Paraoxonase-1 Controversy, *Circulation: Cardiovascular Interventions* (2011) 4:401-404

Karaz′niewicz-Łada, M., Danielak, D., et al., HPLC–MS/MS method for the simultaneous determination of clopidogrel, its carboxylic acid metabolite and derivatized isomers of thiol metabolite in clinical samples, *Journal of Chromatography B* (2012) 911: 105– 112

Kazui, M., Nishiya, Y., et al., Identification of the human cytochrome P450 enzymes involved in the two oxidative steps in the bioactivation of clopidogrel to its pharmacologically active metabolite, *Drug Metab. Dispos.* (2010) 38(1): 92-9

Ksycinska, H., Rudzki, P., et al., Determination of clopidogrel metabolite (SR26334) in human plasma by LC-MS, *J. Pharm. Biomed. Anal.*, (2006) 41:533– 539

Lagorce, P., Perez, Y., et al., Assay method for the carboxylic acid metabolite of clopidogrel in human plasma by gas chromatography-mass spectrometry, *J. Chromatogr. B* (1998) 720:107-117

Lainesse, A., Ozalp, Y., et al., Bioequivalence study of clopidogrel bisulfate film-coated tablet, *Arzneimittelforschung*. (2004) 54:600-4

Mitakos, A., Panderi, I., Determination of the carboxylic acid metabolite of clopidogrel in human plasma by liquid chromatography-electrospray ionization mass spectrometry, *Anal. Chim. Acta*, (2004) 50:107–114

Nirogi, V. S., Kandikere, N., et al., Quantification of clopidogrel in human plasma by sensitive liquid chromatography/tandem mass spectrometry, *Rapid Commun. Mass Spectrom.* (2006) 20:1695–1700

Patent application EP 2540729 A1: (7aS, 2'S)-2-2-oxo-clopidogrel as anti-thrombotic compound

Robinson, A., Hillis, J., et al., The validation of a bioanalytical method for the determination of clopidogrel in human plasma, *Journal of Chromatography B*, (2007) 848:344–354

Savi, P., Pereillo, J. M., et al., Identification and Biological Activity of the Active Metabolite of Clopidogrel, *Thromb. Haemost.* (2000) 84: 891–6

Silvestro, L., Gheorghe, M. C., et al. Development and validation of an HPLC–MS/MS method to determine clopidogrel in human plasma. Use of incurred samples to test back-conversion., *Journal of Chromatography B*, (2010) 878: 3134–3142

Silvestro, L., Gheorghe, M. C., et al. Development and validation of an HPLC–MS/MS method to quantify clopidogrel acyl glucuronide, clopidogrel acid metabolite, and clopidogrel in plasma samples avoiding analyte back-conversion, *Analitical and Bioanalitical Chemistry* (2011) 401(3):1023-34

Shuldiner, A. R., O'Connell, J. R., et al., Association of cytochrome P450 2C19 genotype with the antiplatelet effect and clinical efficacy of clopidogrel therapy., *Journal of the American Medical Association* 302(8) (2009)849-57

Takahashi, M., Pang, H., et al., Quantitative determination of clopidogrel active metabolite in human plasma by LC–MS/MS, *Journal of Pharmaceutical and Biomedical Analysis* (2008) 48:1219–1224

Taubert, D., Kastrati, A., et al., Pharmacokinetics of clopidogrel after administration of a high loading dose, *Thromb. Haemost.* (2004) 92(2): 311-6.

Taubert, D., von Beckerath, N., et al., Impact of P-glycoprotein on clopidogrel absorption, *Clin. Pharmacol. Ther.* (2006) 80(5):486-501

Von Beckerath, N., Taubert, D., et al., Absorption, Metabolization, and Antiplatelet Effects of 300-, 600-, and 900-mg Loading Doses of Clopidogrel, *Circulation.* (2005) 112: 2946-2950

Yerino, P., Toren, P., Ogilvie, B., Parkinson, A. (2006) *Poster presentation. 14th North American Regional ISSX Meeting.*

Available at http://mms.technologynetworks.net/posters/0324.pdf. Accessed 04 Feb. 2011

Yousef, A. M., Diab, O., Pharmacokinetics of 600mg loading dose of clopidogrel in patients undergoing percutaneous coronary intervention, *AJPP* (2013) 7(11):574-584

Zhang, H., Lau, W. C., et al., Formation Of The Thiol Conjugates And Active Metabolite of Clopidogrel By Human Liver Microsomes, *Molecular Pharmacology Fast Forward* (2012)

Zhu, H. J., Wang, X., et al., Carboxylesterase 1 as a determinant of clopidogrel metabolism and activation, *The Journal of Pharmacology and Experimental Therapeutics - Fast Forward*, Published on December 28, (2012)

In: Clopidogrel
Editors: J. P. Alesci and A. Victorino
ISBN: 978-1-62948-336-8
© 2014 Nova Science Publishers, Inc.

Chapter 4

FROM MECHANISM TO THERAPEUTICS: OVERCOMING INTER-INDIVIDUAL VARIABILITY IN CLOPIDOGREL THERAPY

Haoming Zhang* and Paul F. Hollenberg
Department of Pharmacology,
The University of Michigan Medical School, Ann Arbor, MI, US

ABSTRACT

Clopidogrel is widely used to treat acute coronary syndromes (ACS) and peripheral vascular diseases, particularly among patients undergoing percutaneous coronary intervention (PCI). It is the therapeutic agent of choice to prevent thrombotic events associated with cardiovascular stenting. However nearly 20-40% patients respond poorly to the standard regimen of clopidogrel therapy and these patients are at increased risk for ischemic complications and cardiovascular deaths. Although there are intensive efforts to search for genetic markers for this interindividual variability in clopidogrel therapy, results have been mixed and inconclusive. Based on the mechanistic studies of clopidogrel metabolism, it is most likely that the interindividual variability in clopidogrel therapy is multifactorial. A crucial factor contributing to the variable response to clopidogrel is that clopidogrel is a prodrug requiring

* Corresponding author: Haoming Zhang, PhD, Department of Pharmacology, The University of Michigan Medical School, 1150 West Medical Center Drive, 2220A MSRB III, Ann Arbor, MI 48109-5632, Tel: 734-764-6182, Fax: 734-763-5387, E-mail: haom@umich.edu.

bioactivation to the active metabolite by hepatic cytochrome P450 enzymes (CYPs or P450s). P450s are inherently polymorphic and the activities of P450s are prone to induction and inhibition by numerous xenobiotics. Furthermore, extensive metabolism of clopidogrel in the liver primarily by P450s through multiple pathways leads to the formation of multiple metabolites, which significantly attenuate the formation of the active metabolite. These attrition pathways likely exacerbate the problems of the variable response. To overcome the interindividual variability, efforts have been made to mitigate the metabolic attritions as exemplified in the development of prasugrel, vicagrel, and reversible antithrombotic agents such as ticagrelor, cangrelor and elinogrel. We took a mechanistic approach to investigate the metabolism of clopidogrel by human liver microsomes (HLMs). Our results demonstrated that formation of mixed disulfide conjugates between the active metabolite of clopidogrel and thiol reductants is an integral part of the bioactivation process in the liver. Furthermore, we found that mixed disulfide conjugates of clopidogrel are capable of releasing the active metabolite in the presence of glutathione without the need for P450-mediated bioactivation. Results from *ex vivo* studies using platelet-rich plasma revealed that these stable mixed disulfide conjugates of clopidogrel inhibit platelet aggregation when induced by adenosine diphosphate (ADP) agonist. Inhibition of platelet aggregation without the requirement of bioactivation by P450s holds great promise to overcome the interindividual variability in clopidogrel therapy.

ABBREVIATION

ACS	acute coronary syndromes
ADP	adenosine diphosphate
CPT	6-chloropyridazine-3-thiol
CYP	cytochrome P450
DFT	2,5-dimethylfuran-3-thiol
HLMs	human liver microsomes
IPA	inhibition of platelet aggregation
LC-MS/MS	liquid chromatography tandem mass spectrometry
LOF	loss of function
NPT	3-nitropyridine-2-thiol
PCI	percutaneous coronary intervention
PD	pharmacodynamics
PK	pharmacokinetics

PPP	platelet-poor plasma
PRP	platelet-rich plasma.

Introduction

Platelet activation and aggregation play important roles in cardiovascular diseases or atherothrombosis. Activation of platelets due to sheer arterial pressure or plaque rupture resulting from progressive build-up of plaque can trigger a cascade of signaling events that facilitate the formation of thrombus and eventual thrombogenesis. These events are generally accompanied with complete blockage of arteries leading to ischemia or cardiovascular deaths. Antithrombotic drugs are widely used to prevent the formation of thrombi, especially in the early stage of the thrombogenesis, by disrupting some of the key signaling pathways.

Aspirin and clopidogrel are two of the most widely used antithrombotic drugs. Aspirin inhibits cyclooxygenase 1 and thereby prevents formation of thromboxane A2, while clopidogrel is an antagonist of the $P2Y_{12}$ receptor and inhibits adenosine diphosphate (ADP)-induced platelet aggregation. Clopidogrel belongs to a class of thienopyridine antithrombotic drugs that also include ticlopidine (first generation) and prasugrel (third generation) (see Figure 1). The three thienopyridine antithrombotic drugs share the same mechanism of action on $P2Y_{12}$; they irreversibly modify cysteine residues of the receptor to prevent ADP-induced platelet aggregation. In this review, we focus our efforts on the use of clopidogrel as an antithrombotic agent and recent advances made to overcome the interindividual variability associated with clopidogrel.

Pharmacokinetics (PK) and Metabolism of Clopidogrel

Clopidogrel was launched in the United States in 1998 for the treatment of coronary artery and peripheral artery diseases. Its superior efficacy to aspirin was first demonstrated in the CAPRIE study [1], a large clinical trial that involved 19185 patients. Results from the CAPRIE study showed that long-term administration of clopidogrel to patients with atherosclerotic vascular disease was more effective than aspirin in reducing the combined risk of ischemic stroke, myocardial infarction, or vascular death. Specifically, patients treated with clopidogrel had an annual combined risk of 5.32% compared with that of 5.83% for patients on aspirin. It was also noted in the CAPRIE study that the overall safety profile of clopidogrel was at least as good as aspirin. The common side effects of clopidogrel included rash, diarrhea, upper gastrointestinal discomfort, intracranial haemorrhage and gastrointestinal haemorrhage. In the CLASSICS study, the safety of clopidogrel was compared with that of ticlopidine [2]. Patients with successful stent placement were randomized to receive either clopidogrel or ticlopidine in combination with aspirin. The results showed that the safety and tolerability of clopidogrel were superior to those of ticlopidine; clopidogrel was well tolerated even at a loading dose (LD) of 300 mg with no increased risk of bleeding.

These and other clinical trials established that clopidogrel is a superior antithrombotic drug to aspirin and ticlopidine. Serious, potentially life-threatening side effects associated with ticlopidine were largely mitigated, such as hyponatremia, nephritic syndrome, hepatotoxicity, neutropenia and thrombocytopenia. Since launched to market, clopidogrel has gained widespread use with annual sales worth more than $6 billion in 2009 and 2010. Dual antiplatelet therapy with clopidogrel in combination with aspirin has become the gold standard to treat patients with ACS or undergoing PCI. The American Heart Association and American College of Cardiology guidelines recommend the dual antiplatelet therapy for all PCI patients before and after the procedure [3].

The major drawback associated with clopidogrel therapy is the great variability in the pharmacodynamic response. It has been well documented that approximately 20-40% patients do not respond to clopidogrel. To better understand the pharmacological responses to clopidogrel, a large number of basic and clinical studies have been carried out in the past two decades. Increasing evidence suggests that the interindividual variability in clopidogrel therapy is closely related with the metabolism of clopidogrel. An overview of the metabolic pathways of clopidogrel is shown in Figure 2, which is a composite from a number of pharmacokinetic and metabolic studies.

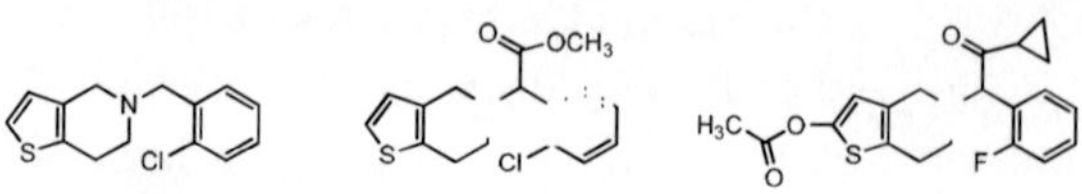

Ticlopidine Clopidogrel Prasugrel

Figure 1. Chemical structures of three thienopyridine antithrombotic drugs: ticlopidine, clopidogrel, and prasugrel.

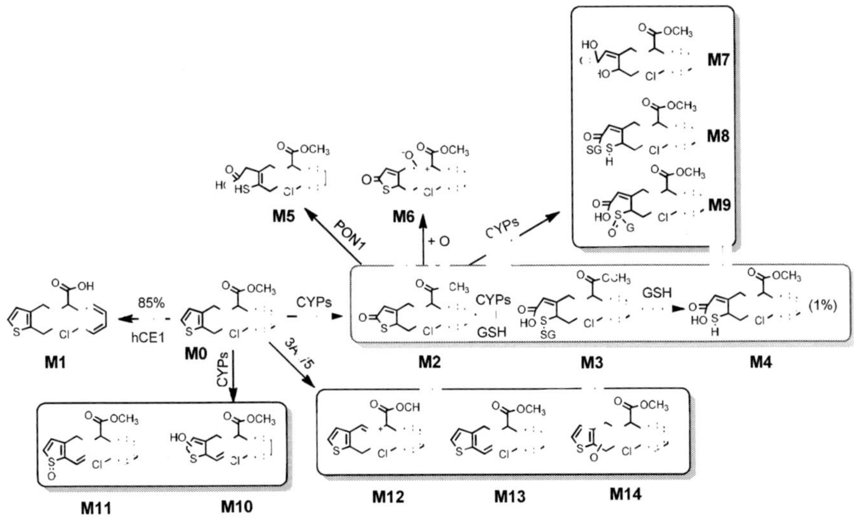

Figure 2. Overall metabolic pathways for clopidogrel. The bioactivation follows the pathway of M0→M2→M3→M4. hCE1 is human carboxylesterase 1.

Early PK studies in human subjects suggested that clopidogrel was extensively metabolized; clinical studies did not show any detectable amount of clopidogrel in plasma [4]. The major circulating compound was the inactive carboxylic acid, M1, which constituted 85% of injested clopidogrel. Within 1 hour of oral administration of 75 mg clopidogrel, M1 reached a C_{max} of 2.8 mg/ml. It seemed that clopidogrel was rapidly absorbed in the small intestine and hydrolyzed by human carboxylesterase 1 (hCE1) to give rise to M1 [5]. This rapid absorption seemed contradictory to the slow onset time for the inhibition of platelet aggregation (IPA); significant inhibition of platelet aggregation was usually achieved between 3 to 7 days of dosing at 75 mg/day or 6 hours after a LD of 300 mg [6].

The disposition of clopidogrel was investigated using radiolabeled ^{14}C-clopidogrel [7]. It was found that clopidogrel was excreted in both urine and feces. Consistent with the results reported by Caplain et al. [4], a C_{max} was reached within 1 hour of oral administration. However, the half-life for plasma elimination of radiolabeled compounds was found in the range of 14-28 days, indicative of irreversible binding of the radiolabeled compounds to protein targets. Recently, a more sensitive liquid chromatography tandem mass spectrometric [LC-MS/MS] method was developed to directly determine the PK of the active isomer of M4 [8]. It was found that a C_{max} of 38.5 ng/ml was achieved within one hour of administration of a 300 mg LD in healthy subjects. This confirmed that clopidogrel is rapidly absorbed and metabolized.

The important role of hepatic metabolism for clopidogrel was established by the seminal work of Savi and coworkers [9, 10]. It was found that clopidogrel was completely ineffective in hepatectomized rats after oral or intravenous administration. Furthermore, a global CYP inhibitor, SKF525-A, dramatically decreased the anti-aggregating effect of clopidogrel. These results suggested that clopidogrel is a prodrug requiring biotransformation to the pharmacologically active metabolite, M4, by hepatic P450s.

Our current understanding of the bioactivation process of clopidogrel can be largely attributed to in vitro studies of biotransformation of clopidogrel by human liver microsomes (HLMs). The generally accepted bioactivation mechanism of clopidogrel involves a two-step bioactivation process as depicted in Figure 2. In the first step, clopidogrel is oxidized by the P450s to form a thiolactone metabolite, M2, or 2-oxoclopidogrel and in the second step, M2 is further oxidized by P450s to give the M4. The first study that elucidated the chemical structure of the M4 was reported by Pereillo et al. [11]. Structural analysis using LC-MS/MS, ^{1}H and ^{13}C NMR revealed that the M4 is 2-{1-[1-(2-chlorophenyl)-2-methoxy-2-oxoethyl]-4-sulfanyl-3-piperidinylidene}acetic acid, which contains a reactive sulfhydryl group. Furthermore, the authors determined the stereochemistry of the M4 as having the S configuration at C7 and the Z configuration at the double bond between C3-C16. It was found that incubation of human platelet-rich plasma (PRP) with M4 prevented binding of ^{33}P-2MeS-ADP to platelets. Furthermore, incubation of human PRP with the M4 inhibited platelet aggregation induced by the ADP agonist. The IC_{50} values for the inhibition of the ^{33}P-2MeS-ADP binding and of the platelet aggregation were 0.53 and 1.8 μM, respectively. The comparable IC_{50} values demonstrated that the two events were closely related.

Obviously, both steps in the bioactivation require the participation of P450s (see Figure 2). The contributions of specific isoforms of P450s to each step of the biotransformation were determined by the use of specific monoclonal antibodies and selective chemical inhibitors for each of the P450 isoforms [12]. It was found that CYP1A2, 2B6 and 2C19 play major roles in the catalytic oxidation of clopidogrel to 2-oxoclopidogrel, and CYP2B6, 2C9, 2C19 and 3A4 contributed most to the second step of the bioactivation. It is evident that CYP2C19 and 2B6 participate in both steps of the bioactivation. Elucidation of the chemical mechanism for the conversion of 2-oxoclopidogrel to the M4 can be largely credited to the original work of Dansette and coworkers [13-15]. According to the proposed mechanism shown in Figure 3,

2-oxoclopidogrel is first oxidized at the thiophene sulfur to form an S-oxide intermediate that is then readily hydrolyzed to give rise to the sulfenic acid intermediate, M-SOH.

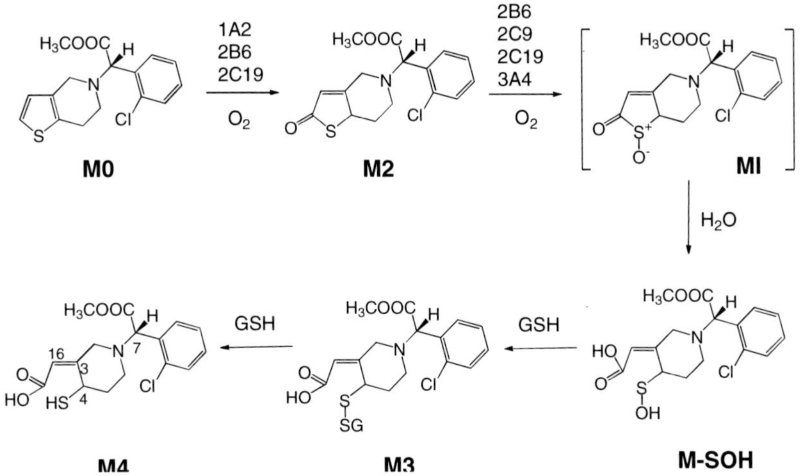

Figure 3. Generally accepted mechanism for bioactivation of clopidogrel to the active metabolite. This mechanism is based on the studies of Dansette and coworkers [13, 14].

The sulfenic acid intermediate is subsequently reduced by GSH to form the mixed disulfide conjugate, M3. The M3 glutathionyl conjugate then rapidly exchanges with another molecule of GSH to generate the M4 active metabolite. This mechanism is supported by the observation that GSH is required for production of the M4 in HLMs [11, 12, 16]. Due to high levels of endogenous GSH in the human liver, it is conceivable that this rapid thiol-exchange reaction would readily occur in humans. A controversial proposal suggested that paraoxonase 1 [PON1] is responsible for production of the M4 in humans [17]. PON1, an endogenous esterase expressed in humans, catalyzes hydrolysis of ester bonds to yield both an acid and alcohol. It was argued that hydrolysis of the thiol ester bond of 2-oxoclopidogrel directly by PON1 gives rise to M4. This controversy has been recently resolved through detailed mechanistic studies of the catalytic reactions leading to the formation of M4 by Dansette and coworkers [15, 18]. Based on detailed structural analyses of the products formed by both PON1 and HLMs, it was concluded that PON1 is responsible for the formation of an *endo* isomer of the active metabolite M4, denoted as M5 in Figure 2. The M5 *endo* isomer has no antiplatelet activity and thus it is not expected to elicit antithrombotic activity in vivo. In fact, metabolism of 2-oxoclopidogrel in the absence of PON1 inhibitor demonstrated that production of M4 by P450s is the major bioactivation pathway while production of the *endo* isomer M5 is a minor metabolic pathway [15].

As noted above, clopidogrel is extensively metabolized in humans. In addition to the bioactivation pathway leading to the formation of M4, many attrition pathways exist. As illustrated in Figure 2, clopidogrel is prone to oxidative biotransformation at multiple sites. In particular, the thiophene and piperidine rings are vulnerable to oxidation. It is known that oxidative biotransformation of thiophene by P450s leads to formation of the thiophene S-oxide and thiophene epoxides [19-21]. Formation of these reactive, electrophilic intermediates is associated with the toxic effects of thiophenes, at least in some cases [22, 23]. In the biotransformation of clopidogrel, oxidation of the thiophene motif gives rise to thiophene S-oxide and the hydroxylated products M10 and M11, while oxidation of the piperidine motif leads to the pyridinium and monooxygenated products, M12-M14. The latter pathway is primarily mediated by CYP3A4/5 [24]. Studies of the metabolism of ticlopidine in rats identified the glutathionyl conjugate of ticlopidine S-oxide as the main biliary metabolite [25]. A recent study characterized the mechanism by which the thiolactone ring opening occurred and identified the novel byproducts, M7-M9, resulting from deactivation of the MI intermediate (see Figure 3] [26]. Taking into account many of the attrition pathways, Zhu and Zhou [26] estimated that the overall yield for bioactivation of clopidogrel to the M4 is approximately 1%. This great attrition in the metabolic bioactivation of clopidogrel not only reduces the efficacy of clopidogrel, but also generates significant amounts of unwanted reactive byproducts that are potentially toxic.

A number of studies have demonstrated that reactive metabolites produced during the metabolism of clopidogrel and ticlopidine inactivate P450s and modify protein targets. In particular, it was suggested that the idiosyncratic events of agranulocytosis and cholestatic hepatitis associated with the use of ticlopidine may result from the production of reactive metabolites and the subsequent binding of these reactive metabolites to cellular targets [27-30]. Richter and coworkers reported that clopidogrel and ticlopidine are potent mechanism-based inhibitors of CYP2B6 [31]. It was later reported that the mechanism-based inhibition of CYP2B6 by clopidogrel was attributed to both destruction of the heme and covalent modification of CYP2B6 proteins [32]. It was found that the M4 active metabolite formed a disulfide bond with Cys 475 located in a putative substrate access channel, and it was also postulated that a reactive metabolite, likely either an S-oxide or epoxide, was responsible for the modification of the heme. Ha-Duong and coworkers have reported selective mechanism-based inhibition of CYP2C19 by ticlopidine [33, 34]. These authors suggested that the inhibition of CYP2C19 was due to modifications of the protein by reactive metabolites of ticlopidine such as ticlopidine S-oxide. A comparative study by Nishiya et al. was carried out to differentiate the mechanism-based inhibition of human CYP2B6 by three thienopyridine drugs, ticlopidine, clopidogrel and prasugrel [35]. A similar study by the same group compared the inhibitory effects [IC_{50}] of the thienopyridines and the respective thiolactones and active metabolites on the catalytic activities of multiple human P450 isozymes [36]. It was found that: [1] ticlopidine and clopidogrel inhibit CYP2B6 with IC_{50} of 0.051 and 0.018 μM, respectively, and CYP2C19 with IC_{50} of 0.20 and 0.52 μM, respectively [3]. Ticlopidine also inhibits CYP2D6 with an IC_{50} of 0.35 μM [4]. Prasugrel and its thiolactone metabolite are weak inhibitors. Although there are no reports relating clopidogrel to idiosyncratic toxicity, inhibition of CYP2B6 and 2C19 may result in drug-drug interactions. It was also reported that coadministration of clopidogrel or ticlopidine with bupropion, an anti-smoking drug primarily metabolized by CYP2B6, significantly inhibited the metabolism of bupropion [37]. The drug-drug interactions of clopidogrel with proton pump inhibitors have been extensively investigated. Results from a number of studies supported the notion that coadministration of omeprazole decreases the effectiveness of clopidogrel due to inhibition of CYP2C19 by omeprazole [38-40]. A recent study investigated the effect of omeprazole on the active metabolite in healthy human subjects using a sensitive LC-MS/MS approach [8]. The study convincingly showed that coadministration of omeprazole led to a significant decrease in the active isomer of clopidogrel.

Pharmacodynamic Response to Clopidogrel

It is now known that the pharmacological target of clopidogrel is a platelet ADP receptor, referred to as $P2Y_{12}$ receptor. The $P2Y_{12}$ receptor is located on the surface of platelets and belongs to a group of G protein-coupled purinergic receptors. Upon activation by the ADP agonist, it couples with the α subunit of G protein to down regulate adenylyl cyclase. A cascade of events that follow the binding of ADP induce platelet activation and the subsequent activation of glycoprotein (GP) IIb/IIIa complex resulting in platelet aggregation and endothelial adherence. It was found that clopidogrel elicits its pharmacological effects through covalent modification of cysteine residues of the P2Y_{12} receptor. It was first reported that the active metabolite of clopidogrel forms disulfide bonds with free thiols of Cys17 and Cys 270 of the P2Y_{12} receptor based on site-directed mutagenesis in combination with the use of the thiol reagent *p*-chloromercuribenzene sulfonic acid [41]. Cys 17 and Cys 270 were thought to be located at the N-terminus and in the third extracellular loop respectively, not close to the ADP binding site. A subsequent study of the interaction of the active metabolite of prasugrel, R-138727, raised doubts that Cys 17 and Cys 270 are the sites of the reaction. Rather, it concluded that Cys 97 (upper portion of the predicted third transmembrane region) and Cys 175 (second extracellular loop) are irreversibly modified by R-138727 [42]. These two cysteine residues form an intramolecular disulfide bond close to the ADP binding site. From a chemical standpoint of view, it is unlikely that the nucleophilic sulfhydryl group of the active metabolite of clopidogrel or prasugrel reacts with nucleophilic free thiols of cysteine. It is most likely that the sulfhydryl group of the M4 active metabolite exchanges thiols with the Cys97-Cys175 disulfide bond, leading to the irreversible modification.

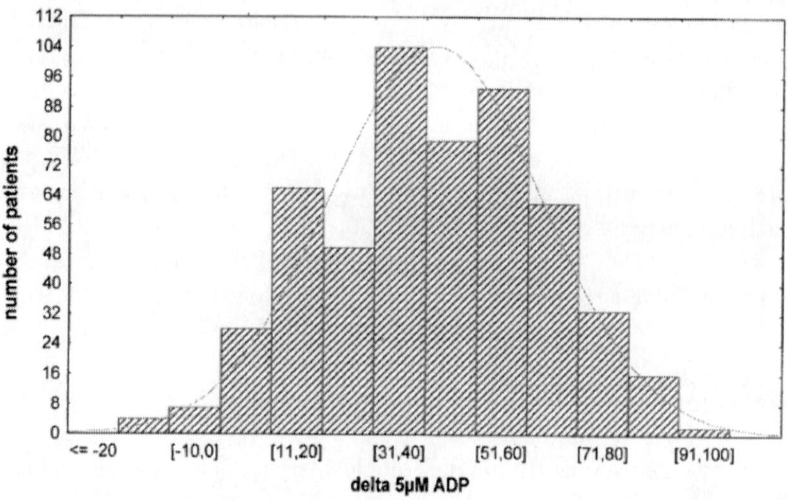

Figure 4. Distribution of changes in 5 μmol of adenosine diphosphate [ADP]-induced platelet aggregation in 544-patients after receiving clopidogrel therapy. Negative changes in aggregation values represent aggregation values after the administration of clopidogrel that were higher than the baseline readings. This figure was reprinted from ref [47] with permission from the Elsevier Publishing Company.

Irreversible inhibition of the $P2Y_{12}$ receptor by clopidogrel is consistent with the pharmacological response to clopidogrel, which is characterized by a slow onset time and lasting effects of several days in humans. It was observed that inhibition of platelet aggregation reaches steady state in 3 to 5 days after oral administration at a daily dose of 75 mg. This slow onset time of clopidogrel likely results from the highly inefficient bioactivation process. It seems that accumulative inhibition of platelets by the M4 active metabolite is necessary to reach a steady-state pharmacological response. Since modification of the $P2Y_{12}$ receptor is irreversible, the pharmacodynamic response to clopidogrel lasts until new platelets are generated.

Although the onset time of clopidogrel at a maintenance dose (MD) of 75 mg is slow, it was found that a 300 mg LD prior to the MD significantly shortened the pharmacological response [6]. The antithrombotic effect of a 300 mg LD within 6 hours was comparable to that achieved after a few days of MD, demonstrating that beneficial effects of a loading dose in effective prevention of thrombosis as early as possible.

A number studies have demonstrated the effectiveness of clopidogrel, especially used in combination with aspirin, in preventing reoccurrence of thrombosis in ACS or PCI patients [43-45]. One major problem associated with clopidogrel therapy has persisted till now. That is the interindividual variability in the pharmacological response to clopidogrel. It was noted in as early as 2003 that responses of patients to clopidogrel were markedly different. Gurbel and coworkers [46] reported that 31% of the patients who underwent elective coronary stenting after receiving aspirin (325 mg) and clopidogrel (300 LD and 75 mg MD) for five days did not respond to the antithrombotic therapy. The IPAs observed in these patients were significantly less. In a large heterogeneous population, it was found that the response to clopidogrel determined as ex vivo platelet aggregation showed a wide range of variability that followed a normal, bell-shaped distribution [47] (also see Figure 4). The mean and standard deviation were 41.9% and 20.8%, respectively, and the bell-shaped distribution was slightly shifted to non-responders on the left. Approximately 19% of the patients exhibited an IPA of ≤20%. The clinical importance of this finding has been demonstrated in a number of clinical studies [46, 48-51]. It was reported that 5-11% of PCI-patients were non-responders [IPA < 10%] and might correspond to recurrence of thrombotic ischemic complications [51]. Matetzky et al. correlated the nonresponsiveness to post-stent ischemic events and showed that 25% of PCI-patients were resistant to clopidogrel and these patients had higher risks for recurrent cardiovascular events [49]. A similar result was reported for patients undergoing non-emergent stenting [48].

Since Gurbel et al. reported the variable response to clopidogrel [46], numerous studies have been reported which attempted to identify the factor(s) that cause the variability in responses and to find solutions to overcome this interindividual variability. Although several genetic markers such as *CYP2C19*, *ABCB1* (the gene encoding for the drug efflux transporter p-glycoprotein), *P2Y*$_{12}$, and *ITG3* (the gene encoding the β-subunit of GPIIb/IIIa) were suggested, only the association of *CYP2C19* with the interindividual variability was positive. The association of clopidogrel response variability with *CYP2C19* was first reported by Hulot et al. in 2006 [52]. It was found that the pharmacodynamic response to clopidogrel in 28 healthy male volunteers treated with clopidogrel at a 75 mg MD for 7 days correlated significantly with the *CYP2C19* genotype. Specifically, the *CYP2C19*2* loss-of-function (LOF) allele was associated with a marked decrease in platelet responsiveness to clopidogrel. Further studies extended this pharmacogenetic study to a number of P450s including *CYP1A2, 2B6, 2C19, 2C9, 3A4 and 3A5* [53, 54]. It was found that common LOF polymorphisms of *CYP2C19* and *2C9* were associated with decreased levels of the active metabolite of clopidogrel, but not with prasugrel, and the decreased level of the active metabolite is correlated with poorer pharmacodynamic responses [53]. Simon et al. attempted to associate the genotypes of *CYP3A5, CYP2C19, ABCB1*, *P2Y*$_{12}$, and *ITGB3* with clinical outcomes after acute myocardial infarction [55]. The authors correlated the allelic variants of the aforementioned genes of 2208 patients presenting with acute myocardial infarction and receiving clopidogrel therapy with the risk of death during one year of follow-up. It was found that patients carrying *CYP2C19* LOF alleles had a higher rate of subsequent cardiovascular events than those who did not. A genome wide association study (GWAS) of 429 healthy Amish persons revealed that *CYP2C19*2* LOF gene was associated with diminished platelet response to clopidogrel treatment and poorer cardiovascular outcomes. However, *CYP2C19*2* LOF gene accounted for only 12% of the variation in platelet aggregation induced by the ADP agonist. Thus, it is likely that the inter-individual variability is multifactorial. Systematic meta-analyses of large populations of patients to assess the association of the *CYP2C19 LOF* gene with ischemic outcomes reaffirmed that *CYP2C19* LOF was a major risk factor for nonresponsiveness to clopidogrel [56, 57]. Of 11959 patients, carriers of *CYP2C19*2* displayed a 30% increase in the risk of major cardiovascular events compared with non-carriers [56]. However, it is noteworthy that other clinical studies did not show any correlation between *CYP2C19*2* and the outcomes of clopidogrel treatment [58, 59].

OVERCOMING INTERINDIVIDUAL VARIABILITY

It is well documented that pharmacodynamic responses to clopidogrel differ significantly among different groups of patients. Many factors have been suggested to account for this variable response including ethnicity, age, obesity, drug-drug interactions, compliance, metabolic attritions, etc. In spite of extensive studies, overcoming the variability in the response is still a critically important area of research and development. Therefore, we review here the main progress in this area.

Genetic Testing

A large body of evidence supports the notion that the *CYP2C19* genotype correlates with the decreased bioactivation of clopidogrel and an increased risk for adverse cardiovascular events. This correlation seems to justify genetic testing to identify patients homozygous/heterozygeous for the *CYP2C19* LOF genotype so that adjustments in dosage can be made or alternative antithrombotic drugs can be used for these patients. Recently, a decision analysis was carried out to evaluate the cost-effectiveness of a *CYP2C19*2* genotype-guided strategy of antiplatelet therapy in ACS patients undergoing PCI [60]. Three scenarios of decision making were considered in this study: 1]. treat all patients with clopidogrel without genetic testing. 2] treat all patients with prasugrel without genetic testing. 3]. perform genetic testing and treat subjects with the *CYP2C19*2* genotype with prasugrel and wild-type subjects with clopidogrel. The results suggested that a genotype-guided strategy was only marginally beneficial over empiric approaches. A meta-analysis of the data from 14 clinical trials involving 19601 patients was performed to evaluate the role of clinical testing for *CYP2C19* and *ABCB1* polymorphisms [61]. Although the study confirmed the association of the *CYP2C19*2* polymorphism with increased risk for adverse cardiovascular events in coronary artery patients treated with clopidogrel, it concluded that this association had such low predictive value that it did not justify routine genetic testing. The low predictive value for genetic testing of the *CYP2C19* genotype likely results from many confounding factors contributing to the effectiveness of clopidogrel. Furthermore, results from the GWAS study showed that the *CYP2C19*2* genotype accounts for only ~12% of the variable responses [62]. In addition, there is a wide range of variability observed under various conditions, as summarized by Gurbel and Tantry [63], which makes it impractical to perform routine genetic testing. However, genetic testing may be cost-effective in a targeted sub-population of patients. For example, it was reported that a genetically guided antiplatelet therapy strategy may be cost-effective for ACS patients of Pacific Islanders who have high prevalence (45%) of the *CYP2C19*2* genotype [64].

Elimination of Metabolic Attrition and Bioactivation

Based on extensive studies of the PK/PD of clopidogrel, it is understood that metabolism of clopidogrel by hepatic P450s is one of the major determinants that cause the interindividual variability, as well as to some extent the related toxicity. The association of the *CYP2C19*2* genotype with clopidogrel therapy boils down to a metabolic activation problem. Therefore, to overcome the interindividual variability, it would be desirable to reduce metabolic attrition or eliminate the requirement for metabolic activation. In line with this consideration, researchers continue formulating new strategies to develop $P2Y_{12}$ antagonists with better efficacy and consistency.

A good example is the successful development of prasugrel, the third generation of thienopyridine antithrombotic drug launched to the market in 2009. Compared with the chemical structure of clopidogrel, the structure of prasugrel differs with respect to two key motifs as shown in Figure 3: 1] the methoxy group of clopidogrel is replaced with a cyclopropyl group in prasugrel. This modification eliminates the major attrition pathway to form inactive carboxylic acid; and 2]. an acetoxy group is attached to the C2 of the thiophene ring, which allows facile formation of the thiolactone intermediate through hCE2 without the requirement for bioactivation by P450s. These modifications significantly improve the PK/PD parameters, leading to rapid absorption and metabolism of prasugrel in the small intestine by CYP3A4/5. The efficacy of prasugrel is not associated with the CYP genotypes. In the TRITON-TIMI 38 trial [65] and a subsequent substudy [66], it was found that prasugrel results in greater IPA and is more effective for the prevention of ischemic events than clopidogrel in ACS patients. The improved effectiveness of prasugrel over clopidogrel is largely attributed to the elimination of the pathways leading to metabolic attrition based on two pieces of evidence: 1]. In vitro studies showed that the active metabolites of clopidogrel and prasugrel were equipotent in inhibiting platelet aggregation [67]; and 2]. In vivo studies showed that prasugrel was 10-fold more potent than clopidogrel at inhibiting ex vivo platelet aggregation [68]. These results suggest that the efficacy for bioactivation of prasugrel is significantly higher than that of clopidogrel due to the elimination of a major metabolic attrition pathway. As illustrated in the case of prasugrel, elimination of metabolic attritions greatly increases the efficacy of antithrombotic therapy. Prasugrel is certainly an alternative antithrombotic drug for patients who are nonresponsive to clopidogrel therapy. However, the high cost and increased risks for bleeding in elderly patients may limit its use.

In an analogous approach to prasugrel, vicagrel was prepared by adding an acetoxy group to the C2 of clopidogrel. Therefore, the thiolactone of clopidogrel was produced by hCE2 rather than by oxidative biotransformation mediated by P450s. Results from preclinical studies showed that the levels of the thiolactone intermediate generated from vicagrel were six times higher than those from clopidogrel and that vicagrel was as potent as prasugrel in rats. The authors anticipated that vicagrel would have better efficacy and more consistent pharmacodynamic response than clopidogrel.

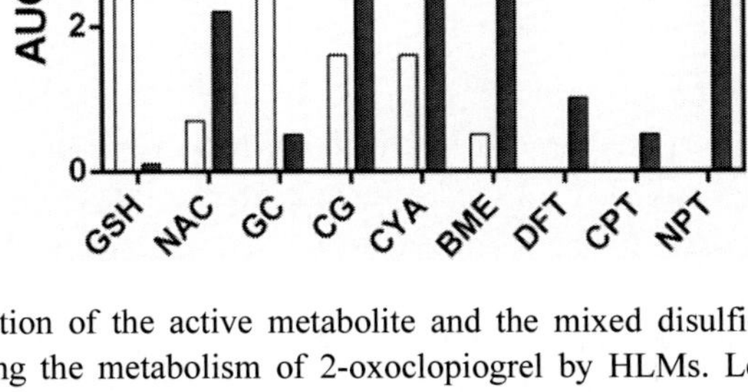

Figure 5. Formation of the active metabolite and the mixed disulfide conjugates of clopidogrel during the metabolism of 2-oxoclopiogrel by HLMs. Legend: open bar, active metabolite [AM]; solid bar, mixed disulfide conjugates of clopidogrel. GSH, NAC, GC, CG, CYA, BME, DFT, CPT and NPT stand for glutathione, N-acetyl-L-cysteine, γ-L-glutamyl-L-cysteine, Cys-Gly, β-mercaptoethanol, cysteamine, 2,5-dimethylfuran-3-thiol, 6-chloropyridazine-3-thiol, and 3-nitropyridine-2-thiol, respectively. This figure is reprinted from Figure 3 of ref [69] with permission from *Molecular Pharmacology*.

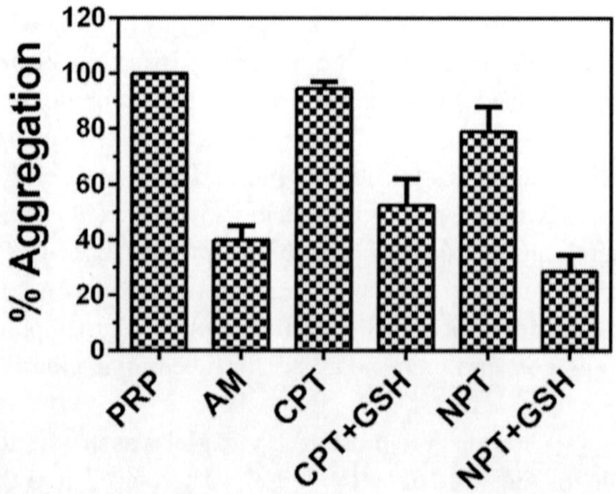

Figure 6. Inhibition of platelet aggregation in platelet-rich plasma [PRP] by the active metabolite released from the CPT and NPT conjugates. The released AM were incubated with PRP at 37 °C for 60 min followed by the addition of 10 μM ADP agonist. Platelet aggregation was then measured with light transmission aggregometry. This figure is adapted from Figure 7 of ref [69] permission from *Molecular Pharmacology*.

Although metabolic attrition is mitigated in prasugrel and vicagrel, many of the attrition pathways associated with the second step of the bioactivation, as shown in Figure 2, remain. Thus, a critical question is whether it is possible to deliver the active metabolites of the thienopyridines in the complete absence of oxidative biotransformation.

Our recent findings of stable mixed disulfide conjugates of clopidogrel make this a possibility. Under normal circumstances, glutathione (GSH) is present at high concentrations (1-5 mM) in the metabolic reactions of clopidogrel, which is required to produce the M4 active metabolite. As such formation of the mixed disulfide conjugate of clopidogrel is negligible and thus it evades detection and detailed characterization. We reasoned that if the bioactivation of clopidogrel proceeds in two distinct steps as shown in Figure 3, metabolism of clopidogrel in the presence of thiol reductants with high redox potentials would be expected to produce the mixed disulfide conjugates as terminal products without formation of the M4 active metabolite. This was exactly what we observed during the metabolism of clopidogrel by HLMs in the presence of various thiol reductants (16, 69]. As shown in Figure 5, formation of the M4 active metabolite was greatly affected by the thiol compound used. In the presence of 2,5-dimethylfuran-3-thiol (DFT],

6-chloropyridazine-3-thiol (CPT) and 3-nitropyridine-2-thiol (NPT), only the mixed disulfide conjugates were observed without any detectable M4 active metabolite. These observations strongly support the mechanism proposed by Dansette et al. [13, 15] (see Figure 3). We also observed that the mixed disulfide conjugates were readily reduced by GSH to release the M4 active metabolite. Furthermore, the mixed disulfide conjugates exhibited ex vivo antiplatelet activity in the presence of GSH as shown in Figure 6. These findings provide a platform to quantitatively generate the M4 active metabolite without the need for bioactivation by P450s. This platform also eliminates all the metabolic attrition pathways leading to formation of unwanted byproducts except for the hCE2 pathway resulting in formation of the inactive carboxylic acid metabolite. Rapid release of the active metabolite from the conjugates in the presence of GSH is also well suited for the development of the conjugates as intravenous form of antithrombotic agents with fast onset time. Therefore, the use of thienopyridine conjugates as antithrombotic agents is a viable approach to overcome the interindividual variability in response to clopidogrel therapy. This approach starts with a known drug with a proven record of efficacy and safety profiles. In addition, high levels of GSH concentrations (1-10 mM) in the liver and in the blood allow for facile thiol exchange between GSH and the conjugates. Therefore, the conjugates of thienopyridines offer unique advantages over thienopyridine drugs by eliminating the defects of parent drugs while retaining the effective components. More importantly, production of the M4 active metabolite does not require bioactivation by P450s and is not affected by P450-mediated drug-drug interactions or toxicity. Use of the conjugates as antithrombotic agents is one step further toward the elimination of the metabolic attrition and the requirement for bioactivation by P450s. This is a promising approach to overcome the interindividual variability.

It is of note that a new class of $P2Y_{12}$ antagonists have been developed as reversible antithrombotic agents including ticagrelor, cangrelor and elinogrel. Structurally they differ completely from thienopyridines. Although inhibiting ADP-induced platelet aggregation, they do not covalently modify the $P2Y_{12}$ receptor. Therefore, they exhibit fast onset time for IPA as well as fast offset time once withdrawn. Ticagrelor, a cyclopentyl-triazolo-pyrimidine, was approved in July 2011 by the Food and Drug Administration (FDA) as an antithrombotic drug to treat ACS. In the PLATO study (a large phase III clinical trial), ticagrelor was found to be more effective than clopidogrel in reducing mortality [70]. A negative impact on major bleeding in some patients and an increased frequency of dyspnea were noted [71]. The decision by the

FDA to approve ticagrelor was questioned citing lack of clinical efficacy and safety [72]. It remains to be seen whether ticagrelor plays a major role in antithrombotic therapy. Cangrelor is an adenosine triphosphate (ATP) analog acting on the $P2Y_{12}$ receptor that has been developed for intravenous use only. It has very short half-life [73]. Results from early and interim clinical trials were negative. A new trial, CHAMPION PHONIX trial, is currently under way. Elinogrel, a sulphonylurea derivative, is in phase II clinical trials and it is being developed as both an oral and an intravenous agent. Its efficacy and safety remains to be seen.

CONCLUSION

Since launched to the market in 1998, clopidogrel has become one of the most successful antithrombotic drugs. Dual therapy with clopidogrel and aspirin is now the gold standard to treat patients with ACS and undergoing PCI. The efficacy and safety profiles of clopidogrel therapy validate that $P2Y_{12}$ is a good drug target for the inhibition of platelet aggregation. Tremendous progress has been made in the past two decades to understand the pharmacokinetics and pharmacodynamics of clopidogrel and of thienopyridines as antithrombotic drugs in general. Based on this information, alternative strategies are now formulated to overcome the primary drawbacks of clopidogrel, in particular the inter-individual variability in the pharmacodynamic responses. It is evident that the drawbacks of clopidogrel stem largely from metabolic activation and attrition. Prasugrel, vicargrel, and mixed disulfide conjugates of thienopyridines offer promising solutions. These alternatives retain the covalently aspect of modifying the $P2Y_{12}$ receptor, rendering the characteristic lasting effects of IPA. Reversible antagonists of $P2Y_{12}$ offer rapid on/off-set times and may be useful for defined relatively limited periods of time according to clinical need. At present, the benefit of genetic testing to guide clopidogrel therapy is unclear because the cost-effectiveness is marginal. With continuous efforts to develop the next generations of antithrombotic agents with better efficacy and consistency, genotype-guided clopidogrel strategies may not be necessary in the future.

REFERENCES

[1] CAPRIE Steering Committee (1996). A randomised, blinded, trial of clopidogrel versus aspirin in patients at risk of ischaemic events (CAPRIE). CAPRIE steering committee, *Lancet*, *348*, 1329-1339.

[2] Bertrand, M. E., Rupprecht, H. J., Urban, P., Gershlick, A. H. & Investigators, C. (2000). Double-blind study of the safety of clopidogrel with and without a loading dose in combination with aspirin compared with ticlopidine in combination with aspirin after coronary stenting : The clopidogrel aspirin stent international cooperative study (CLASSICS), *Circulation*, *102*, 624-629.

[3] King, S. B., 3rd, Smith, S. C., Jr., Hirshfeld, J. W., Jr., Jacobs, A. K., Morrison, D. A., Williams, D. O., Writing Committee, M., Feldman, T. E., Kern, M. J., O'Neill, W. W., Schaff, H. V., Whitlow, P. L., Adams, C. D., Anderson, J. L., Buller, C. E., Creager, M. A., Ettinger, S. M., Halperin, J. L., Hunt, S. A., Krumholz, H. M., Kushner, F. G., Lytle, B. W., Nishimura, R., Page, R. L., Riegel, B., Tarkington, L. G. & Yancy, C. W. (2008). 2007 focused update of the ACC/AHA/SCAI 2005 guideline update for percutaneous coronary intervention: A report of the American College of Cardiology/American Heart Association task force on practice guidelines: 2007 writing group to review new evidence and update the ACC/AHA/SCAI 2005 guideline update for percutaneous coronary intervention, writing on behalf of the 2005 writing committee, *Circulation*, *117*, 261-295.

[4] Caplain, H., Donat, F., Gaud, C. & Necciari, J. (1999). Pharmacokinetics of clopidogrel, *Semin. Thromb. Hemost. 25 Suppl 2*, 25-28.

[5] Tang, M., Mukundan, M., Yang, J., Charpentier, N., LeCluyse, E. L., Black, C., Yang, D., Shi, D. & Yan, B. (2006). Antiplatelet agents aspirin and clopidogrel are hydrolyzed by distinct carboxylesterases & clopidogrel is transesterificated in the presence of ethyl alcohol, *J Pharmacol Exp Ther*, *319*, 1467-1476.

[6] Cadroy, Y., Bossavy, J. P., Thalamas, C., Sagnard, L., Sakariassen, K. & Boneu, B. (2000). Early potent antithrombotic effect with combined aspirin and a loading dose of clopidogrel on experimental arterial thrombogenesis in humans, *Circulation*, *101*, 2823-2828.

[7] Lins, R., Broekhuysen, J., Necciari, J. & Deroubaix, X. (1999). Pharmacokinetic profile of ^{14}C-labeled clopidogrel, *Semin. Thromb. Hemost. 25 Suppl*, *2*, 29-33.

[8] Tuffal, G., Roy, S., Lavisse, M., Brasseur, D., Schofield, J., Delesque Touchard, N., Savi, P., Bremond, N., Rouchon, M. C., Hurbin, F. & Sultan, E. (2011). An improved method for specific and quantitative determination of the clopidogrel active metabolite isomers in human plasma, *Thromb. Haemost.*, *105*, 696-705.

[9] Savi, P., Combalbert, J., Gaich, C., Rouchon, M. C., Maffrand, J. P., Berger, Y. & Herbert, J. M. (1994). The antiaggregating activity of clopidogrel is due to a metabolic activation by the hepatic cytochrome P450-1A, *Thromb. Haemost.*, *72*, 313-317.

[10] Savi, P., Herbert, J. M., Pflieger, A. M., Dol, F., Delebassee, D., Combalbert, J., Defreyn, G. & Maffrand, J. P. (1992). Importance of hepatic metabolism in the antiaggregating activity of the thienopyridine clopidogrel, *Biochem Pharmacol*, *44*, 527-532.

[11] Pereillo, J. M., Maftouh, M., Andrieu, A., Uzabiaga, M. F., Fedeli, O., Savi, P., Pascal, M., Herbert, J. M., Maffrand, J. P. & Picard, C. (2002). Structure and stereochemistry of the active metabolite of clopidogrel, *Drug Metab Dispos*, *30*, 1288-1295.

[12] Kazui, M., Nishiya, Y., Ishizuka, T., Hagihara, K., Farid, N. A., Okazaki, O., Ikeda, T. & Kurihara, A. (2010). Identification of the human cytochrome P450 enzymes involved in the two oxidative steps in the bioactivation of clopidogrel to its pharmacologically active metabolite, *Drug Metab Dispos*, *38*, 92-99.

[13] Dansette, P. M., Libraire, J., Bertho, G. & Mansuy, D. (2009). Metabolic oxidative cleavage of thioesters: Evidence for the formation of sulfenic acid intermediates in the bioactivation of the antithrombotic prodrugs ticlopidine and clopidogrel, *Chem. Res. Toxicol.*, *22*, 369-373.

[14] Dansette, P. M., Thebault, S., Bertho, G. & Mansuy, D. (2010). Formation and fate of a sulfenic acid intermediate in the metabolic activation of the antithrombotic prodrug prasugrel, *Chem. Res. Toxicol.*, *23*, 1268-1274.

[15] Dansette, P. M., Rosi, J., Bertho, G. & Mansuy, D. (2012). Cytochromes P450 catalyze both steps of the major pathway of clopidogrel bioactivation, whereas paraoxonase catalyzes the formation of a minor thiol metabolite isomer, *Chem. Res. Toxicol.*, *25*, 348-356.

[16] Zhang, H., Lau, W. C. & Hollenberg, P. F. (2012). Formation of the thiol conjugates and active metabolite of clopidogrel by human liver microsomes, *Mol Pharmacol.*, *82*, 302-309.

[17] Bouman, H. J., Schomig, E., van Werkum, J. W., Velder, J., Hackeng, C. M., Hirschhauser, C., Waldmann, C., Schmalz, H. G., ten Berg, J. M. & Taubert, D. (2011). Paraoxonase-1 is a major determinant of clopidogrel efficacy, *Nat Med*, *17*, 110-116.

[18] Dansette, P. M., Rosi, J., Bertho, G. & Mansuy, D. (2011). Paraoxonase-1 and clopidogrel efficacy, *Nat Med.*, *17*, 1040-1041; author reply 1042-1044.

[19] Dansette, P. M., Thang, D. C., el Amri, H. & Mansuy, D. (1992). Evidence for thiophene-S-oxide as a primary reactive metabolite of thiophene in vivo: Formation of a dihydrothiophene sulfoxide mercapturic acid, *Biochem Biophys Res Commun.*, *186*, 1624-1630.

[20] Dalvie, D. K., Kalgutkar, A. S., Khojasteh-Bakht, S. C., Obach, R. S. & O'Donnell, J. P. (2002). Biotransformation reactions of five-membered aromatic heterocyclic rings, *Chem Res Toxicol.*, *15*, 269-299.

[21] Dansette, P. M., Bertho, G. & Mansuy, D. (2005). First evidence that cytochrome P450 may catalyze both S-oxidation and epoxidation of thiophene derivatives, *Biochem Biophys Res Commun.*, *338*, 450-455.

[22] Beaune, P., Dansette, P. M., Mansuy, D., Kiffel, L., Finck, M., Amar, C., Leroux, J. P. & Homberg, J. C. (1987). Human anti-endoplasmic reticulum autoantibodies appearing in a drug-induced hepatitis are directed against a human liver cytochrome P-450 that hydroxylates the drug, *Proc Natl Acad Sci U S A. 84*, 551-555.

[23] O'Donnell, J. P., Dalvie, D. K., Kalgutkar, A. S. & Obach, R. S. (2003). Mechanism-based inactivation of human recombinant P450 2C9 by the nonsteroidal anti-inflammatory drug suprofen, *Drug Metab Dispos.*, *31*, 1369-1377.

[24] Zhu, Y. & Zhou, J. (2012). Identification of the significant involvement and mechanistic role of CYP3A4/5 in clopidogrel bioactivation, *ACS Med Chem Lett.*, *3*, 844-849.

[25] Shimizu, S., Atsumi, R., Nakazawa, T., Fujimaki, Y., Sudo, K. & Okazaki, O. (2009). Metabolism of ticlopidine in rats: Identification of the main biliary metabolite as a glutathione conjugate of ticlopidine S-oxide, *Drug Metab Dispos.*, *37*, 1904-1915.

[26] Zhu, Y. & Zhou, J. (2012). In vitro biotransformation studies of 2-oxo-clopidogrel: Multiple thiolactone ring-opening pathways further attenuate prodrug activation, *Chem Res Toxicol.*, *26*, 179-190.

[27] Love, B. B., Biller, J. & Gent, M. (1998). Adverse haematological effects of ticlopidine. Prevention, recognition and management, *Drug Saf.*, *19*, 89-98.

[28] Ono, K., Kurohara, K., Yoshihara, M., Shimamoto, Y. & Yamaguchi, M. (1991). Agranulocytosis caused by ticlopidine and its mechanism, *Am. J. Hematol.*, *37*, 239-242.

[29] Skurnik, Y. D., Tcherniak, A., Edlan, K. & Sthoeger, Z. (2003). Ticlopidine-induced cholestatic hepatitis, *Ann. Pharmacother.*, *37*, 371-375.

[30] Mizushima, M., Iwata, N., Fujimoto, T. T., Ishikawa, K. & Fujimura, K. (2005). Patient characteristics in ticlopidine hydrochloride-induced liver injury: Case-control study, *Hepatology*, *33*, 234-240.

[31] Richter, T., Murdter, T. E., Heinkele, G., Pleiss, J., Tatzel, S., Schwab, M., Eichelbaum, M. & Zanger, U. M. (2004). Potent mechanism-based inhibition of human CYP2B6 by clopidogrel and ticlopidine, *J Pharmacol Exp Ther.*, *308*, 189-197.

[32] Zhang, H., Amunugama, H., Ney, S., Cooper, N. & Hollenberg, P. F. (2011). Mechanism-based inactivation of human cytochrome P450 2B6 by clopidogrel: Involvement of both covalent modification of cysteinyl residue 475 and loss of heme, *Mol Pharmacol.*, *80*, 839-847.

[33] Ha-Duong, N. T., Dijols, S., Macherey, A. C., Dansette, P. M. & Mansuy, D. (2001). Inhibition by ticlopidine and its derivatives of human liver cytochrome P450. Mechanism-based inactivation of CYP2C19 by ticlopidine, *Adv Exp Med Biol.*, *500*, 145-148.

[34] Ha-Duong, N. T., Dijols, S., Macherey, A. C., Goldstein, J. A., Dansette, P. M. & Mansuy, D. (2001). Ticlopidine as a selective mechanism-based inhibitor of human cytochrome P450 2C19, *Biochemistry*, *40*, 12112-12122.

[35] Nishiya, Y., Hagihara, K., Ito, T., Tajima, M., Miura, S., Kurihara, A., Farid, N. A. & Ikeda, T. (2009). Mechanism-based inhibition of human cytochrome P450 2B6 by ticlopidine, clopidogrel & the thiolactone metabolite of prasugrel, *Drug Metab Dispos.*, *37*, 589-593.

[36] Hagihara, K., Nishiya, Y., Kurihara, A., Kazui, M., Farid, N. A. & Ikeda, T. (2008). Comparison of human cytochrome P450 inhibition by the thienopyridines prasugrel, clopidogrel & ticlopidine, *Drug Metab Pharmacokinet*, *23*, 412-420.

[37] Turpeinen, M., Tolonen, A., Uusitalo, J., Jalonen, J., Pelkonen, O. & Laine, K. (2005). Effect of clopidogrel and ticlopidine on cytochrome

P450 2B6 activity as measured by bupropion hydroxylation, *Clin Pharmacol Ther.*, *77*, 553-559.

[38] Gilard, M., Arnaud, B., Cornily, J. C., Le Gal, G., Lacut, K., Le Calvez, G., Mansourati, J., Mottier, D., Abgrall, J. F. & Boschat, J. (2008). Influence of omeprazole on the antiplatelet action of clopidogrel associated with aspirin: The randomized, double-blind OCLA (omeprazole clopidogrel aspirin). study, *J. Am. Coll. Cardiol. 51*, 256-260.

[39] Cuisset, T., Frere, C., Quilici, J., Poyet, R., Gaborit, B., Bali, L., Brissy, O., Morange, P. E., Alessi, M. C. & Bonnet, J. L. (2009). Comparison of omeprazole and pantoprazole influence on a high 150-mg clopidogrel maintenance dose the PACA (proton pump inhibitors and clopidogrel association). prospective randomized study, *J. Am. Coll. Cardiol.*, *54*, 1149-1153.

[40] Juurlink, D. N., Gomes, T., Ko, D. T., Szmitko, P. E., Austin, P. C., Tu, J. V., Henry, D. A., Kopp, A. & Mamdani, M. M. (2009). A population-based study of the drug interaction between proton pump inhibitors and clopidogrel, *CMAJ*, *180*, 713-718.

[41] Ding, Z., Kim, S., Dorsam, R. T., Jin, J. & Kunapuli, S. P. (2003). Inactivation of the human $P2Y_{12}$ receptor by thiol reagents requires interaction with both extracellular cysteine residues, Cys17 and Cys270, *Blood*, *101*, 3908-3914.

[42] Algaier, I., Jakubowski, J. A., Asai, F. & von Kugelgen, I. (2008). Interaction of the active metabolite of prasugrel, R-138727, with cysteine 97 and cysteine 175 of the human $P2Y_{12}$ receptor, *J Thromb Haemost.*, *6*, 1908-1914.

[43] Chen, Z. M., Jiang, L. X., Chen, Y. P., Xie, J. X., Pan, H. C., Peto, R., Collins, R., Liu, L. S. & group, C. c. (2005). Addition of clopidogrel to aspirin in 45,852 patients with acute myocardial infarction: Randomised placebo-controlled trial, *Lancet*, *366*, 1607-1621.

[44] Sabatine, M. S., Cannon, C. P., Gibson, C. M., Lopez-Sendon, J. L., Montalescot, G., Theroux, P., Lewis, B. S., Murphy, S. A., McCabe, C. H. & Braunwald, E. (2005). Effect of clopidogrel pretreatment before percutaneous coronary intervention in patients with ST-elevation myocardial infarction treated with fibrinolytics: The PCI-CLARITY study, *JAMA*, *294*, 1224-1232.

[45] Yusuf, S., Zhao, F., Mehta, S. R., Chrolavicius, S., Tognoni, G. & Fox, K. K. (2001). Effects of clopidogrel in addition to aspirin in patients

with acute coronary syndromes without ST-segment elevation, *N. Engl. J. Med.*, *345*, 494-502.

[46] Gurbel, P. A., Bliden, K. P., Hiatt, B. L. & O'Connor, C. M. (2003). Clopidogrel for coronary stenting: Response variability, drug resistance and the effect of pretreatment platelet reactivity, *Circulation*, *107*, 2908-2913.

[47] Serebruany, V. L., Steinhubl, S. R., Berger, P. B., Malinin, A. I., Bhatt, D. L. & Topol, E. J. (2005). Variability in platelet responsiveness to clopidogrel among 544 individuals, *J. Am. Coll. Cardiol.*, 45, 246-251.

[48] Bliden, K. P., DiChiara, J., Tantry, U. S., Bassi, A. K., Chaganti, S. K. & Gurbel, P. A. (2007). Increased risk in patients with high platelet aggregation receiving chronic clopidogrel therapy undergoing percutaneous coronary intervention: Is the current antiplatelet therapy adequate?, *J. Am. Coll. Cardiol.*, *49*, 657-666.

[49] Buonamici, P., Marcucci, R., Migliorini, A., Gensini, G. F., Santini, A., Paniccia, R., Moschi, G., Gori, A. M., Abbate, R. & Antoniucci, D. (2007). Impact of platelet reactivity after clopidogrel administration on drug-eluting stent thrombosis, *J. Am. Coll. Cardiol.*, *49*, 2312-2317.

[50] Matetzky, S., Shenkman, B., Guetta, V., Shechter, M., Beinart, R., Goldenberg, I., Novikov, I., Pres, H., Savion, N., Varon, D. & Hod, H. (2004). Clopidogrel resistance is associated with increased risk of recurrent atherothrombotic events in patients with acute myocardial infarction, *Circulation*, *109*, 3171-3175.

[51] Muller, I., Besta, F., Schulz, C., Massberg, S., Schonig, A. & Gawaz, M. (2003). Prevalence of clopidogrel non-responders among patients with stable angina pectoris scheduled for elective coronary stent placement, *Thromb. Haemost. 89*, 783-787.

[52] Hulot, J. S., Bura, A., Villard, E., Azizi, M., Remones, V., Goyenvalle, C., Aiach, M., Lechat, P. & Gaussem, P. (2006). Cytochrome P450 2C19 loss-of-function polymorphism is a major determinant of clopidogrel responsiveness in healthy subjects, *Blood*, *108*, 2244-2247.

[53] Brandt, J. T., Close, S. L., Iturria, S. J., Payne, C. D., Farid, N. A., Ernest, C. S., 2nd, Lachno, D. R., Salazar, D. & Winters, K. J. (2007). Common polymorphisms of CYP2C19 and CYP2C9 affect the pharmacokinetic and pharmacodynamic response to clopidogrel but not prasugrel, *J Thromb Haemost*, *5*, 2429-2436.

[54] Frere, C., Cuisset, T., Morange, P. E., Quilici, J., Camoin-Jau, L., Saut, N., Faille, D., Lambert, M., Juhan-Vague, I., Bonnet, J. L. & Alessi, M. C. (2008). Effect of cytochrome P450 polymorphisms on platelet

reactivity after treatment with clopidogrel in acute coronary syndrome, *Am. J. Cardiol.*, *101*, 1088-1093.

[55] Simon, T., Verstuyft, C., Mary-Krause, M., Quteineh, L., Drouet, E., Meneveau, N., Steg, P. G., Ferrieres, J., Danchin, N. & Becquemont, L. (2009). Genetic determinants of response to clopidogrel and cardiovascular events, *N. Engl. J. Med.*, *360*, 363-375.

[56] Hulot, J. S., Collet, J. P., Silvain, J., Pena, A., Bellemain-Appaix, A., Barthelemy, O., Cayla, G., Beygui, F. & Montalescot, G. (2010). Cardiovascular risk in clopidogrel-treated patients according to cytochrome P450 2C19*2 loss-of-function allele or proton pump inhibitor coadministration: A systematic meta-analysis, *J. Am. Coll. Cardiol.*, *56*, 134-143.

[57] Sofi, F., Giusti, B., Marcucci, R., Gori, A. M., Abbate, R. & Gensini, G. F. (2011). Cytochrome P450 2C19*2 polymorphism and cardiovascular recurrences in patients taking clopidogrel: A meta-analysis, *Pharmacogenomics J.*, *11*, 199-206.

[58] Brackbill, M. L., Kidd, R. S., Abdoo, A. D., Warner, J. G., Jr. & Harralson, A. F. (2009). Frequency of CYP3A4, CYP3A5, CYP2C9 and CYP2C19 variant alleles in patients receiving clopidogrel that experience repeat acute coronary syndrome, *Heart Vessels*, *24*, 73-78.

[59] Pare, G., Mehta, S. R., Yusuf, S., Anand, S. S., Connolly, S. J., Hirsh, J., Simonsen, K., Bhatt, D. L., Fox, K. A. & Eikelboom, J. W. (2010). Effects of CYP2C19 genotype on outcomes of clopidogrel treatment, *N. Engl. J. Med.*, *363*, 1704-1714.

[60] Lala, A., Berger, J. S., Sharma, G., Hochman, J. S., Scott Braithwaite, R. & Ladapo, J. A. (2013). Genetic testing in patients with acute coronary syndrome undergoing percutaneous coronary intervention: A cost-effectiveness analysis, *J Thromb Haemost*, *11*, 81-91.

[61] Singh, M., Shah, T., Adigopula, S., Molnar, J., Ahmed, A., Khosla, S. & Arora, R. (2012). *CYP2C19*2/ABCB1-C3435T* polymorphism and risk of cardiovascular events in coronary artery disease patients on clopidogrel: Is clinical testing helpful?, *Indian Heart J.*, *64*, 341-352.

[62] Shuldiner, A. R., O'Connell, J. R., Bliden, K. P., Gandhi, A., Ryan, K., Horenstein, R. B., Damcott, C. M., Pakyz, R., Tantry, U. S., Gibson, Q., Pollin, T. I., Post, W., Parsa, A., Mitchell, B. D., Faraday, N., Herzog, W. & Gurbel, P. A. (2009). Association of cytochrome P450 2C19 genotype with the antiplatelet effect and clinical efficacy of clopidogrel therapy, *JAMA*, *302*, 849-857.

[63] Gurbel, P. A. & Tantry, U. S. (2007). Clopidogrel resistance?, *Thromb. Res.*, *120*, 311-321.

[64] Panattoni, L., Brown, P. M., Te Ao, B., Webster, M. & Gladding, P. (2012). The cost effectiveness of genetic testing for CYP2C19 variants to guide thienopyridine treatment in patients with acute coronary syndromes: A New Zealand evaluation, *Pharmacoeconomics 30*, 1067-1084.

[65] Montalescot, G., Wiviott, S. D., Braunwald, E., Murphy, S. A., Gibson, C. M., McCabe, C. H. & Antman, E. M. (2009). Prasugrel compared with clopidogrel in patients undergoing percutaneous coronary intervention for ST-elevation myocardial infarction (TRITON-TIMI 38): Double-blind, randomised controlled trial, *Lancet*, *373*, 723-731.

[66] Michelson, A. D., Frelinger, A. L., 3rd, Braunwald, E., Downey, W. E., Angiolillo, D. J., Xenopoulos, N. P., Jakubowski, J. A., Li, Y., Murphy, S. A., Qin, J., McCabe, C. H., Antman, E. M. & Wiviott, S. D. (2009). Pharmacodynamic assessment of platelet inhibition by prasugrel vs. clopidogrel in the TRITON-TIMI 38 trial, *Eur. Heart J.*, *30*, 1753-1763.

[67] Sugidachi, A., Ogawa, T., Kurihara, A., Hagihara, K., Jakubowski, J. A., Hashimoto, M., Niitsu, Y. & Asai, F. (2007). The greater in vivo antiplatelet effects of prasugrel as compared to clopidogrel reflect more efficient generation of its active metabolite with similar antiplatelet activity to that of clopidogrel's active metabolite, *J Thromb Haemost*, *5*, 1545-1551.

[68] Sugidachi, A., Asai, F., Ogawa, T., Inoue, T. & Koike, H. (2000). The in vivo pharmacological profile of CS-747, a novel antiplatelet agent with platelet ADP receptor antagonist properties, *Br J Pharmacol.*, *129*, 1439-1446.

[69] Zhang, H., Lauver, D. A., Lucchesi, B. R. & Hollenberg, P. F. (2013). Formation, reactivity, and anti-platelet activity of clopidogrel, *Mol Pharmacol*, *83*, 848-56.

[70] Cannon, C. P., Harrington, R. A., James, S., Ardissino, D., Becker, R. C., Emanuelsson, H., Husted, S., Katus, H., Keltai, M., Khurmi, N. S., Kontny, F., Lewis, B. S., Steg, P. G., Storey, R. F., Wojdyla, D. & Wallentin, L. (2010). Comparison of ticagrelor with clopidogrel in patients with a planned invasive strategy for acute coronary syndromes (PLATO): A randomised double-blind study, *Lancet*, *375*, 283-293.

[71] Wijeyeratne, Y. D., Joshi, R. & Heptinstall, S. (2012). Ticagrelor: A $P2Y_{12}$ antagonist for use in acute coronary syndromes, *Expert Rev Clin Pharmacol.*, *5*, 257-269.

[72] Serebruany, V. L. (2012). Ticagrelor FDA approval issues revisited, *Cardiology*, *122*, 144-147.

[73] Storey, R. F., Oldroyd, K. G. & Wilcox, R. G. (2001). Open multicentre study of the P2T receptor antagonist AR-C69931MX assessing safety, tolerability and activity in patients with acute coronary syndromes, *Thromb. Haemost.*, *85*, 401-407.

In: Clopidogrel
Editors: J. P. Alesci and A. Victorino
ISBN: 978-1-62948-336-8
© 2014 Nova Science Publishers, Inc.

Chapter 5

MANAGEMENT OF CLOPIDOGREL HYPERSENSITIVITY

Henry Siu, Antony Kaliyadan, Kimberly L. Campbell, David L. Fischman, Nicholas Ruggiero, Paul Walinsky and Michael P. Savage [*]
Division of Cardiology, Thomas Jefferson University Hospital, Philadelphia, PA, US

ABSTRACT

Clopidogrel, is a cornerstone of therapy for acute coronary syndromes and the prevention of stent thrombosis after percutaneous coronary intervention. Hypersensitivity reactions to clopidogrel typically develop during the initial weeks of therapy and are severe enough to prompt drug discontinuation in 1 to 2% of patients. However, discontinuation of clopidogrel soon after percutaneous coronary intervention is problematic due to the risk of stent thrombosis. Accordingly, the management of clopidogrel hypersensitivity is of significant clinical importance. Clopidogrel desensitization protocols have been developed with success rates of at least 90%. These conventional desensitization methods require a washout period off of medication to allow the hypersensitivity symptoms to resolve before initiating desensitization. This strategy is undesirable in patients with coronary stents who are at risk for stent thrombosis if clopidogrel is

[*] Corresponding author: E-mail: michael.savage@jefferson.edu.

withheld. Recent novel approaches have been described to treat clopidogrel hypersensitivity without drug interruption. Short-term corticosteroids and/or antihistamines are administered to suppress the hypersensitivity symptoms while facilitating the development of physiologic tolerance as clopidogrel is continued. Even after the antiallergy medications are terminated, successful desensitization is maintained during long-term therapy. Alternative antiplatelet drugs have recently become available but the safety and efficacy of these newer agents as potential substitute therapy for patients with clopidogrel hypersensitivity is yet to be determined.

INTRODUCTION: CLOPIDOGREL METABOLISM AND INDICATIONS

Clopidogrel, the most commonly prescribed antiplatelet therapy worldwide, remains among the best-selling medications in history [1]. Though initially manufactured and patented under the trademark Plavix® (Bristol-Myers Squibb/Sanofi Aventis), the patent expiration of clopidogrel as of May 17, 2012 led to the Food and Drug Administration approval of generic clopidogrel in the United States.

A member of the thienopyridine class of antiplatelet agents, clopidogrel directly inhibits adenosine diphosphate induced platelet aggregation by irreversibly binding the $P2Y_{12}$ receptor. The compound has a multi-step metabolism pathway to transform to its active form. The first stage involves the cytochrome P450 pathway in the liver, specifically the CYP1A2, CYP2B6, CYP2C9, CYP2C19, and CTP3A4 isoforms which convert the pro-drug clopidogrel to 2-oxo-clopidogrel, which remains inactive. The second stage involves PON1-mediated hydrolytic cleavage of the 2-oxo-clopidogrel ring structure to a thiol, the fully active metabolite [2]. The complexity of clopidogrel biometabolism due to genetic polymorphisms of metabolism likely accounts for its varying clinical efficacy in select patient populations [3].

At present, clopidogrel is prescribed for a wide range of cardiovascular indications. One of the more common indications for clopidogrel is in the setting of post-percutaneous coronary intervention (PCI) with stent placement. In the 2011 ACCF/AHA/SCAI PCI Guidelines [4], clopidogrel therapy (including other P2Y12 inhibitors) after stent implantation is recommended for:

- *At least* 12 months in patients receiving a stent, whether bare-metal stent (BMS) or drug-eluting stent (DES) during PCI for acute coronary syndrome (ACS)
- *At least* 12 months in patients receiving DES for a non-ACS indication
- *At least* 1 month and ideally *up to* 12 months in patients receiving BMS for a non-ACS indication.

Package labeling for clopidogrel explicitly states the following indications: reduction of atherothrombotic events in patients with recent myocardial infarction (MI), recent stroke, or established peripheral arterial disease, and acute coronary syndrome (ACS) whether unable angina or non-Q-wave MI (NSTEMI) who are to be managed medically or those who do receive PCI therapy with stenting [5].

Despite its many indications and evidenced based efficacy, use of clopidogrel can lead to potential bleeding complications and drug interactions. In addition to these adverse reactions, the next most common is the development of hypersensitivity reactions, which occur in 4-6% of the population and leads to the discontinuation of the medication in 1-2% of cases [5,6]. The following chapter focuses on the presentation, diagnosis, and treatment of clopidogrel hypersensitivity, along with the implications of alternative or newer medications that can be considered when a patient is deemed allergic to clopidogrel.

PRESENTATION AND INCIDENCE OF CLOPIDOGREL HYPERSENSITIVITY

Allergic reaction to clopidogrel most frequently presents as a mild dermatologic eruption which can occur in up to 6% of patients taking clopidogrel [5,6]. In the vast majority of the cases, skin manifestations include a progressive erythematous, macular, morbilliform rash that originates on the face, chest, or abdomen. There have been severe and systemic hypersensitivity reactions reported which include febrile illness, leukopenia, thrombotic thrombocytopenic purpura (TTP), aplastic anemia, angioedema, serum sickness, systemic inflammatory response syndrome, Stevens-Johnson syndrome, and end-organ injury [5]. The following section will review the most common presentation of clopidogrel hypersensitivity, key discriminators for diagnosis, reported incidence, and proposed pathophysiology.

von Tiehl et al. studied 24 patients between September 2005 and June 2006 who were identified to have clopidogrel hypersensitivity after PCI [7]. Median time to onset of clopidogrel hypersensitivity was 6 days (inter-quartile range 3 to 9 days) from drug exposure in this study. In the majority of cases reported, the pruritic macular erythematous rash began on the face, chest, or abdomen with possible spread and confluence to other areas of the body, including the extremities. Palms and soles were affected in 29% (7 of 24 patients). Pruritis is a common manifestation, but one patient who was studied did not report this.

Campbell et al. identified 25 patients with clopidogrel hypersensitivity, between January 2005 to December 2008, and described a similar chronologic pattern and dermatologic presentation [8]. There was a median onset of rash at 6±2 days. The most common presentation was a pruritic rash starting on the trunk and spreading to the extremities in 20 patients; hives were present in 3, non-pruritic rash in 1, and angioedema in 1 patient. Distribution of time to onset of hypersensitivity symptoms is illustrated in *Figure 1*.

Finally, the most recent series of 62 patients with probable or definite cases of clopidogrel hypersensitivity were followed prospectively by Cheema et al., and revealed a clinical presentation similar to prior studies [9]. There was a similar distribution of distinct dermatologic pattern: generalized, pruritic, exanthematous rash predominantly affecting the trunk with or without involvement of the extremities (49 patients; 79%), focal or symmetric area (10 patients; 16%), 2 with angioedema and 1 urticaria (3 patients; 5%) were observed. These patients had a median onset of 5 days from clopidogrel exposure to symptom development, except for the angioedema/urticaria group who presented at day 1.

Diagnosis and Pathophysiology

The diagnosis of clopidogrel hypersensitivity rests heavily on the clinical suspicion via patient history and the temporal relationship of drug exposure to the onset of physical findings. To date, antibody-based laboratory assays and skin tests for clopidogrel hypersensitivity are neither widely available nor clinically applicable. Nevertheless, similar to other drug reactions, definitive causality can be established with careful observation during clopidogrel discontinuation with a resolution of symptoms and return of symptoms when clopidogrel is re-introduced. This method, however, is likely not practical and most importantly, potentially dangerous in the case of post-PCI patients with stent placement. The ill timed onset of clopidogrel hypersensitivity, manifesting within the first 2 weeks of drug initiation, coincides with the timeframe for highest risk of stent thrombosis.

The majority of stent thrombosis, in bare metal or in drug-eluting stents, occur within the first 30 days after stent placement [10]. Cessation of dual antiplatelet therapy (aspirin and clopidogrel) has remained a strong, independent risk factor in the development of stent thrombosis, a condition which is associated with significant morbidity and mortality [11]. Hence, for patients who require clopidogrel treatment, it is essential that both the diagnosis and treatment of clopidogrel hypersensitivity do not involve the discontinuation of dual antiplatelet therapy.

Furthermore, one should recognize that polypharmacy and other in-hospital exposures may complicate the process of deciphering the causative agent responsible for the allergic reaction. Of note, patients are often started on multiple medications at the time of clopidogrel initiation. For instance, the time of an ACS event is accompanied by initiating anti-anginals, anti-hypertensives, anti-thrombotics, and cholesterol lowering therapies. In addition, allergic reactions to radiographic contrast following PCI and contact dermatitis from hospital linen are among conceivable differential diagnoses of an allergic dermatologic reaction.

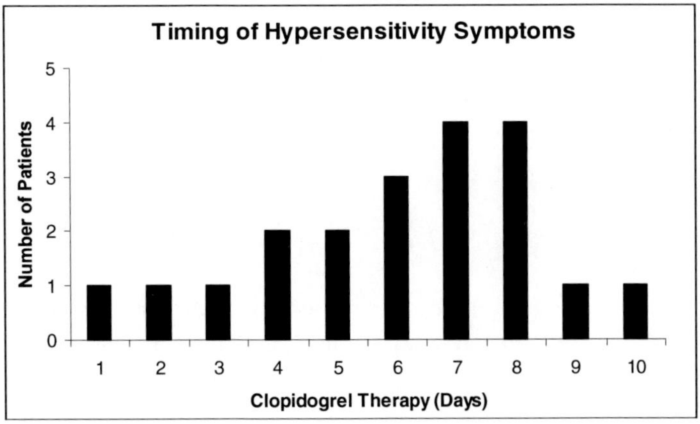

Figure 1. Timing of symptom onset after initiation of drug therapy in 20 patients with clopidogrel hypersensitivity following percutaneous coronary intervention at Thomas Jefferson University Hospital. Note that the incidence peaks at approximately 1 week.

On the basis of signs and symptoms noted in the majority of clopidogrel hypersensitivity cases, a T-cell mechanism has been implicated, but symptoms such as urticaria and angioedema are suggestive of an IgE-mediated immunologic response to an antigen. The elaborate design of the study by Cheema et al. included skin biopsies and cutaneous testing on a portion of patients who completed empiric therapy with steroids and were free of the drug for at least 4 weeks [9]. Seven patients who had generalized skin eruptions and six patients with localized reactions from clopidogrel hypersensitivity underwent skin biopsy and demonstrated the presence of peri-vascular and interstitial lymphocytes with extension into the epidermal layers. Also, patch testing, which could detect delayed reactions, were positive in 34 of 42 studied patients. This data implied a lymphocyte-mediate delayed hypersensitivity response, or Type IV hypersensitivity reaction, which is involved in the majority of clopidogrel hypersensitivity. Three patients who manifested with angioedema/urticaria as the initial presentation of clopidogrel hypersensitivity had a positive response to intra-dermal testing within 30 minutes, suggestive of an immediate hypersensitivity reaction, or Type I hypersensitivity reaction. Notable was that skin prick testing with clopidogrel in this population did not yield any cutaneous reaction, and therefore was not helpful in detecting the potential for a cutaneous allergic reaction [9].

Complete work up of clopidogrel hypersensitivity entails a full-body skin examination, as well as supportive blood work to exclude alternative or additional pathology. The workup may include a complete blood count (CBC) to evaluate for cytopenias, urine analysis, liver function tests, and serum creatinine to detect end organ injury. Skin biopsy should be considered for patients who demonstrate severe dermatologic derangements including toxic epidermal necrolysis syndrome (TENS) and Stevens-Johnson syndrome.

PHARMACOLOGIC ALTERNATIVES TO CLOPIDOGREL

Prevention of stent thrombosis can be achieved with greater degrees of platelet inhibition. As a result, dual antiplatelet therapy with aspirin and $P2Y_{12}$ receptor inhibitor therapy remains the standard of the care post-PCI with stent placement [4]. There are four approved agents currently available: ticlopidine, clopidogrel, prasugrel, and ticagrelor. Historically, ticlopidine, though not referred to in the 2011 ACCF/AHA/SCAI PCI guidelines, is another therapeutic alternative as a $P2Y_{12}$ receptor inhibitor agent. Until recently, outcomes of therapeutic alternatives to clopidogrel have been limited. The following section will discuss the role of ticlopidine, prasugrel, ticagrelor, cilostazol, and warfarin as pharmacologic alternatives to clopidogrel.

Ticlopidine, Prasugrel, Ticagrelor and Cross-Reactivity

Ticlopidine, a first generation thienopyridine, has been proven efficacious in the reduction of bare metal stent thrombosis and preventing cardiovascular events after stroke [12, 13, 14]. There are limited, but positive outcomes for ticlopidine in setting of drug eluting stent placement [15]. Presently, the role for ticlopidine has been minimized compared with the other anti-platelet agents mainly owing to the occurrence of gastrointestinal side effects, neutropenia, thrombocytopenia, and rash. Adverse events with ticlopidine were common in up to 50% of patients ultimately leading to 21% of patients on ticlopidine discontinuing therapy secondary to side effects [12, 14, 16] Neutropenia occurs in 2.4% of patients, with TTP being reported with an incidence of 0.02% [16, 17]. With ticlopidine, CBC is recommended every 2 weeks for the first 3 months of therapy, when hematologic adverse events are most common [16]. Given the significant adverse drug effect profile, the widespread use of ticlopidine has receded with the availability of clopidogrel, which has similar efficacy with fewer side effects.

Cross reactivity between clopidogrel and ticlopidine has been described in several case reports [7, 18, 19, 20]. This could perhaps be due to the chemical similarities between the drugs of this class, as the two compounds differ only by the addition of a carboxymethyl side group (the manufactured ticlopidine is bound to hydrochloride and clopidogrel to bisulfate); the chemical structures of the thienopyridines are shown in *Figure 2*. A large retrospective study on cross-reactivity of these two drugs identified 76 patients who had an allergic or hematologic adverse reaction to either clopidogrel, ticlopidine, or both. Of the 52 patients who had a reaction to clopidogrel, 14 had a reaction to ticlopidine; of the 38 patients who had a reaction to ticlopidine, 14 had a reaction to clopidogrel [21]. This 1 in 4 chance of having a cross-reactivity with ticlopidine is replicated in a skin testing population from the Cheema et al. study of patients with clopidogrel hypersensitivity. In patients who had clopidogrel hypersensitivity, skin testing was positive for allergenic cross-reactivity in 10 of 42 patients (24%) with ticlopidine [9]. All in all, the strategy to manage clopidogrel hypersensitivity via switching to ticlopidine has been attempted, but runs the high risk for cross-reactivity and potentially more serious hematological effects.

In July 2009, the US FDA approved prasugrel, a novel third generation thienopyridine with greater platelet inhibitory function than clopidogrel. In the landmark trial, TRITON-TIMI 38, prasugrel was found to be associated with a statistically significant 19% relative risk reduction in cardiovascular death, nonfatal MI, and nonfatal CVA compared with clopidogrel in patients with STEMI or high-risk ACS/NSTEMI undergoing PCI with stenting (9.9% vs. 12.1%) [22]. The reduction in cardiovascular events in the study was unfortunately counter-balanced by a significant increase in the risk of life-threatening bleeding (1.4% vs. 0.9%). In patients with a history of transient ischemic attack or stroke, the risk of major TIMI bleeds, including intra-cranial hemorrhage, outweighed the benefits of prasugrel. Therefore, the use of prasugrel is contra-indicated in this subgroup of patients. Additional groups at an increased risk for bleeding with prasugrel include patients who are greater than 75 years of age, less than 60 kilograms in weight, and those who have a propensity to bleed or who require the use of other medication that increase the risk of bleeding [23]. However, the TRILOGY-ACS trial of patients with an ACS who did not undergo PCI, medical treatment with prasugrel, compared with clopidogrel, was not demonstrated to be superior in reducing the composite endpoint of CV death, MI and stroke. The heightened platelet inhibition with prasugrel was again associated with increased bleeding [24]. Accordingly, prasugrel remains approved only for patients undergoing PCI in the setting of an ACS.

There have been case reports of patients with clopidogrel hypersensitivity who have been challenged with a different thienopyridine: prasugrel [25, 26, 27]. These single reports describe patients who had presented with various manifestations of clopidogrel hypersensitivity, including the typical rash pattern, angioedema, and even Stevens-Johnson syndrome. The patients all had required thienopyridine following recent PCI implantation, and were switched to prasugrel without complications. These cases illustrate that judicious use of prasugrel, in substitution for selected patients with clopidogrel hypersensitivity, may be practical.

Ticagrelor, approved by the US FDA in July 2011, belongs to a novel chemical class of non-thienopyridine antiplatelet agents, the cyclopentyltriazolopyrimidines. It also differs from clopidogrel and prasugrel in that it binds reversibly, rather than irreversibly, to $P2Y_{12}$ platelet receptor, with a more rapid onset and potent platelet inhibition than clopidogrel. In the PLATO study, 18,624 patients with STEMI and other ACS who were treated with PCI and/or with medical therapy were randomized to ticagrelor or clopidogrel [28]. The results supported the safety and efficacy of this new antiplatelet, with a statistically significant 16% relative risk reduction in the primary end point of composite death from vascular causes, MI, and stroke for patients receiving ticagrelor versus clopidogrel (9.8% vs. 11.7%). While there was no significant difference in the composite rate of major bleeding found between the ticagrelor and clopidogrel groups, there were higher rates of intra-cranial bleeds with ticagrelor. An important distinction of ticagrelor is that it has proven efficacy in patients treated medically for an ACS event without PCI stenting in contrast to prasugrel.

Little is known about the rate of cross-reactivity between clopidogrel and the novel $P2Y_{12}$ receptor inhibitors, both prasugrel and ticagrelor, as patients with a reported allergy to clopidogrel were excluded from enrollment in the large scale TRITON-TIMI 38 and PLATO trials [29, 30]. The chemical structure of prasugrel bears similarities to clopidogrel, whereas ticagrelor, a non-thienopyridine, has a unique chemical configuration. Despite these challenges, data from Cheema et al. did shed some light on this matter [9]. In patients who had clopidogrel hypersensitivity, skin testing was positive for allergenic cross-reactivity in 7 of 42 patients (17%) with prasugrel; cross-reactivity for ticagrelor was not studied.

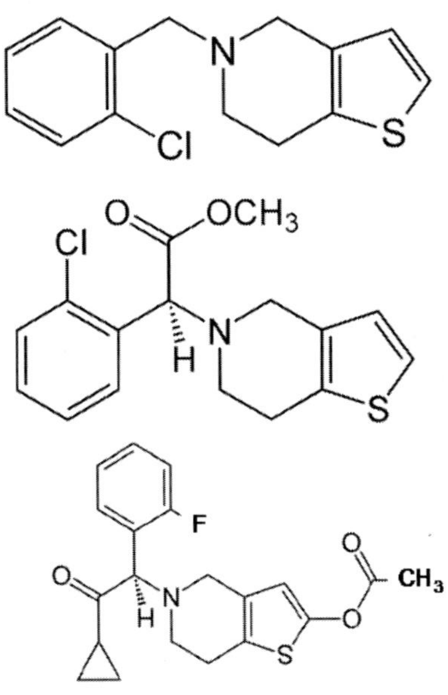

Ticlodipine

Clopidogrel

Prasugrel

Figure 2. Chemical structures of clinically available thienopyridines (Ticlopidine, Clopidogrel, and Prasugrel).

Warfarin

Prior to the advent of novel $P2Y_{12}$ receptor inhibitors, alternatives for additional anti-thrombotic agents have been trialed but have not been adopted into contemporary practice due to a lack of evidence. The use of aspirin in addition to either warfarin or ticlopidine for bare metal stents was evaluated in the FANTASTIC study [31]. This study randomized 485 patients to receive either ticlopidine 250mg twice daily or warfarin adjusted to an international normalized ratio of 2.5 to 3.0 for six weeks following PCI. Compared with ticlopidine, warfarin therapy resulted in a net increase in bleeding complications [21% vs. 13.5%) at 6 weeks, without benefit seen in neither the composite secondary endpoint of death, MI and stent occlusion (8.3% vs. 5.7%) at 6 weeks nor major cardiac clinical events at 6 months. Similarly, a randomized trial of 257 patients assigned to receive antiplatelet therapy (ticlopidine and aspirin) and 260 to receive anticoagulant therapy (intravenous heparin bridge with oral phenprocoumon, and aspirin), demonstrated an increased incidence of both cardiac events and hemorrhagic and vascular complications in the anticoagulation arm [32].

The largest trial, Stent Anticoagulation Restenosis study (STARS), enrolled 1,653 patients receiving bare metal stents and compared aspirin, aspirin with ticlopidine, and aspirin with warfarin for the prevention of a primary end point of stent thrombosis. The primary end point was seen in 3.6%, 2.7%, and 0.5%, respectively, in the three groups. In addition, the group that received aspirin with warfarin had the highest risk of hemorrhagic complications [12]. Although combining aspirin plus warfarin was routinely used prior to the availability of thienopyridines, these trials established that warfarin is inferior to dual antiplatelet therapy in the reduction of cardiovascular events and stent thrombosis following PCI.

Cilostazol

Cilostazol, a phosphodiesterase III inhibitor, has been investigated as a potential alternative and adjunct to thienopyridines. Although a slightly less potent platelet inhibitor, cilostazol is postulated to have pleiotrophic vascular effects including reduction in smooth muscle proliferation and intimal hyperplasia after endothelial injury, which may contribute to more adverse events in the post-PCI period.

Patients receiving bare metal stents were studied in the RACTS trial. In this study, 397 patients were randomly assigned to ticlopidine 250 mg twice daily or cilostazol 100 mg twice daily. At 9 months, there was no significant difference in combined death, MI, stroke or stent thrombosis (32.7% vs 22.9% in ticlopidine vs. cilostazol) [33]. Similarly, a trial randomizing 689 patients to either clopidogrel or cilostazol after BMS placement also demonstrated no statistical difference in the composite incidence of subacute stent thrombosis or major adverse cardiac events at 30 days (2% vs 2.6%, clopidogrel vs. cilostazol, respectively) [34].

There have been limited trials comparing cilostazol with thienopyridines after DES implantation. Park et al., studied 37 patients who received cilostazol post-PCI with paclitaxel DES compared with the 138 patients who received either ticlopidine or clopidogrel post-PCI with paclitaxel DES. There was 1 death and 4 subacute thrombosis vs. 1 non-stent thrombosis related NSTEMI event in the thienopyridine group, respectively [35]. Ahn et al. performed a trial of 280 diabetic patients randomized to either aspirin and cilostazol vs. aspirin and clopidogrel, after 1 month of successful DES stenting with triple anti-thrombotic therapy consisting of aspirin, cilostazol, and clopidogrel. There was no stent thrombosis or MI in either group, but target lesion revascularization (TLR) occurred in 7 cases (5%) in the cilostazol group and 15 cases [10.8%) in the clopidogrel group with mean duration follow up time of 7 months [36].

The totality of available data for cilostazol implicates its potential role in the prevention of stent thrombosis, but effective antiplatelet therapy in the immediate post-PCI period may require a more potent agent. At present, ACCP 2012 guidelines on Antithrombotic therapy recommends that cilostazol 100mg twice daily be used as a substitute for patients who require aspirin and clopidogrel therapy but have an allergy or intolerance to either drug class [37]. However, phosphodiesterase (PDE) 3 inhibitors, such as milirone, which effects increases cyclic AMP for increased cardiac contractility, have been associated with an increased mortality rate in patients with heart failure [38]. Therefore, as a safety precaution, the FDA states that all PDE3 inhibitors including cilostazol, are contraindicated in chronic heart failure of any severity with recognition of increased mortality rates in this group of patients [39].

Vorapaxar

Lastly, vorapaxar is a novel antiplatelet agent that selectively inhibits thrombin-induced platelet activation through antagonism of protease-activated receptor-1 (PAR-1). This agent has not obtained US FDA approval as of 2013, as trials have demonstrated an unacceptable and statistically significant increase in bleeding when used as an additional agent to standard therapy [40, 41]. There have not been large scaled studies directly comparing the efficacy of vorapaxar with other antiplatelet therapies for any cardiovascular indication, and it therefore remains an unclear alternative to clopidogrel.

Clopidogrel Desensitization

Medication desensitization, or the induction of immune tolerance to a medicinal agent, involves repetitive exposures to the allergic inciting agent. The mechanism of drug desensitization has yet to be fully elucidated as mechanisms to the development of immune tolerance remain under investigation. Nevertheless, the leading hypothesis for desensitization involves the induction of antigen-specific mast cell tolerance by gradually increasing the binding of the antigen (the medication) to the IgE receptor without triggering an acute activation of mast cells [42]. Desensitization can be applied for the treatment for Type 1 reactions, but its application has been extended to the management of certain subsets of Type 4 hypersensitivity reactions; these reaction types are often demonstrated in cases of clopidogrel hypersensitivity (see above in section: *Diagnosis and Pathophysiology*). Classic desensitization has been successful in preventing recurrent hypersensitivity manifestations, including anaphylaxis, for agents such as penicillins, cephalosporins, sulfonamides, and aspirin [43, 44]. However, the role of classic desensitization in developing longer-term tolerance to agents that previously caused an adverse hypersensitivity reaction is not well understood, but may be related to a refractory period of mast cell activation that allows for sustained and continued drug dosing [45]. Contraindications to desensitization include Type 2, Type 3, severe cytotoxic Type 4 hypersensitivity reactions of vasculitis or bullous disease such as in Stevens-Johnson Syndrome and TENS, which has been reported in patients who had received clopidogrel. The following section will catalog various published methods of clopidogrel desensitization.

Traditional desensitization protocols have been used with success in patients with clopidogrel hypersensitivity. Table 1 summaries the most commonly cited protocol. These protocols require the withdrawal of clopidogrel to allow hypersensitivity symptoms to resolve prior to the initiation of desensitization. Antihistamines and steroids are withheld for 48-96 hours prior to desensitization, based on the theory that this would better enable the clinician to detect the patient's reaction upon the reintroduction of clopidogrel. Additionally, beta-blockers are withheld, if possible, as a precaution in cases of anaphylaxis requiring treatment with epinephrine. While early reports suggested that beta-blocker therapy is a risk factor for death associated with anaphylaxis in patients undergoing medication desensitization, subsequent analyses portrayed this paradigm as more of theory than reality [46]. Patients are administered escalating doses of clopidogrel starting at 0.005-0.02mg which are doubled every 15-30 minutes until the target dose of 75mg is achieved. If hypersensitivity symptoms recur during desensitization, symptoms are treated and the protocol is held until the symptoms resolve. The protocol is resumed by repeating the inciting dose. The entire desensitization protocol is generally completed within 3-8 hours.

Table 1. Clopidogrel Desensitization Protocol

Dose	Time [h:min]	Desensitizing dose [mg]	Solution concentration	mL
1	0:00	0.005	0.5mg/mL	0.01
2	0:30	0.01	0.5mg/mL	0.02
3	1:00	0.02	0.5mg/mL	0.04
4	1:30	0.04	0.5mg/mL	0.08
5	2:00	0.08	0.5mg/mL	0.16
6	2:30	0.16	0.5mg/mL	0.32
7	3:00	0.3	0.5mg/mL	0.60
8	3:30	0.6	0.5mg/mL	1.20
9	4:00	1.2	5mg/mL	0.24
10	4:30	2.5	5mg/mL	0.5
11	5:00	5	5mg/mL	1
12	5:30	10	5mg/mL	2
13	6:00	20	5mg/mL	4
14	6:30	40	5mg/mL	8
15	7:00	75	75mg tablet	-

Table 1. Finely crushed clopidogrel tablet is dissolved in a compounding agent such as Ora-Plus (Paddock Laboratories Inc., MN, USA) or ethanol

solvent. Each 75mg of clopidogrel is diluted to 150mL with sterile water to make the 0.5mg/mL solution, or to 15mL solution. Adapted from [7, 19].

The first case report of successful clopidogrel desensitization was presented at the American College of Allergy, Asthma, and Immunology Annual Meeting in 2004 (MA, USA). Vigo et al. described the case of a patient who experienced a typical clopidogrel hypersensitivity rash on day five of clopidogrel therapy [47]. Skin testing was performed, suggesting an allergic reaction to clopidogrel and the patient was successfully desensitized with escalating doses of clopidogrel starting at 0.02mg and administered every 15 minutes.

The first reported series of clopidogrel desensitization was by Camara and Almeda [48]. They successfully desensitized three patients using an 8 hour protocol starting at 0.005mg clopidogrel and administering escalating doses of clopidogrel every 30 minutes. Two of the three patients in this case-series had experienced hypersensitivity with both clopidogrel and ticlopidine, necessitating desensitization. Following an identical protocol, Lee-Wong et al. was able to reproduce their success with clopidogrel desensitization on an additional patient [49]. All subsequent desensitization protocols, prior to our report, have been modifications derived from the protocols described by Vigo et al. or Camara and Almeda.

Walker et al. described successful experiences in eight patients with a more rapid 3 hour clopidogrel desensitization protocol [50]. Based on the findings of Vigo et al., they initiated desensitization with a dose of 0.02mg and administered escalating twofold dosages at 15 minute intervals in an intensive care unit setting. Four patients required desensitization for a planned PCI, while the remainder had recent DES placement as their indication for requiring clopidogrel therapy. In contrast to prior desensitization protocols which restricted treatment to patients with cutaneous manifestations of hypersensitivity, this study included two patients experiencing the more severe hypersensitivity reaction of angioedema. Of note, patients had their clopidogrel temporarily discontinued prior to the initiation of the desensitization process.

The largest published case series utilizing and supporting the use of the protocol described by Camara and Almeda studied 24 consecutive patients with clopidogrel hypersensitivity following DES implantation, who subsequently underwent clopidogrel desensitization [7]. In light of the subjects' recent DES implantation and hypersensitivity weighed against the risk for acute stent thrombosis, the patients had clopidogrel discontinued but bridged through a 5 day washout period prior to the desensitization protocol using ticlopidine, a thienopyridine similar in structure to clopidogrel and a conventional agent at that period of time (the study enrolled patients from 2005 to 2006). 20 patients underwent desensitization as an outpatient. Initial desensitization was successful in all patients, with four out of the 24 patients (17%) requiring treatment for cutaneous reactions during the protocol. Two patients (8%) required repeat desensitization - one for persistent rash and another for recurrent rash following 3 days of clopidogrel non-adherence. Limitations to the practical methodology in the study included the 5 day washout period with ticlopidine, which has the potential risk for cross-reactivity as well as risk for side effects due to ticlopidine. Since von Tiehl et al. case series was published, additional case reports have continued to demonstrate the overall success and safety of this desensitization protocol [51, 52].

MANAGEMENT OF HYPERSENSITIVITY REACTION WITHOUT CLOPIDOGREL INTERRUPTION

A treatment strategy for a hypersensitivity reaction to clopidogrel without necessitating the interruption of clopidogrel therapy is an ideal approach with regards to decreasing the risk for adverse cardiac events, especially in patients with recent PCI and stent implantation [53]. In a retrospective analysis from our institution, 25 patients 62 +/- 9 years of age were identified who experienced clopidogrel hypersensitivity following bare metal or drug-eluting stent implantation [8]. The most common symptom was a pruritic maculopapular rash, similar to that observed by von Tiehl et al. [7]. One patient presenting with angioedema was also included. 76% of patients were male, and there was a high prevalence of other atopic illnesses, including 60% reporting an allergy to another drug. A total of 12% presented with STEMI, and 48% present with a NSTEMI/ACS. In total, 16 of the 25 patients received at least one drug-eluting stent.

In a novel approach, patients were treated for their hypersensitivity reactions without interrupting clopidogrel therapy. The treatment regimen included antihistamines alone in five patients, corticosteroids alone in five patients and a combination of antihistamines and corticosteroids in 15 patients. The most commonly prescribed corticosteroid regimen was a 6-day solumedrol taper (Medrol Dosepak®, Pfizer, NY, USA), with the mean corticosteroid therapy duration being 10±8 days (range: 6-30 days). Treatment of clopidogrel hypersensitivity with antihistamines and a short-course of corticosteroids was successful in 22 patients (88%) with majority of patients successfully treated as outpatients (72%). Three patients were treated in a monitored telemetry setting prior to being discharged from their index hospitalization. The patient with angioedema was monitored in the intensive care unit for re-challenge, owing to the life-threatening nature of his previous reaction. Two patients experienced symptom recurrence. Both patients were successfully treated with a longer corticosteroid taper and the leukotrine inhibitor, montelukast, which blocks leukotriene-mediated neutrophil chemotaxis and inflammation.

Three patients in whom desensitization was unsuccessful included one with angioedema, one with rash progressing to desquamation, and one with intolerable pruritis. The patient with angioedema was able to complete a full course of dual antiplatelet therapy with ticlopidine. The patient with desquamation had previously experienced an adverse reaction to ticlopidine, and was treated with aspirin monotherapy. Finally, the patient with pruritis completed 3 weeks of therapy after a bare metal stent, before being treated with aspirin alone.

Patients who were successfully treated were able to continue on clopidogrel in the long term in order to complete the minimum recommended duration of therapy without drug interruption. The mean duration of clopidogrel therapy in these patients was 388±272 days, with 843 days being the longest duration of uninterrupted clopidogrel therapy. There were no cases of stent thrombosis, death, MI, or stroke during treatment or follow-up in the successfully treated patients. The three patients who were unable to tolerate clopidogrel therapy fortunately experienced no stent thrombosis, death, MI, or stroke on alternative treatments.

Cheema et al. also supported a similar treatment strategy of "treating through" clopidogrel hypersensitivity with oral steroids without clopidogrel discontinuation [9]. They followed 62 patients diagnosed with either probable or definite clopidogrel hypersensitivity who were prescribed a 3 week steroid taper, along with diphenhydramine for pruritus if present. All patients were able to continue clopidogrel without interruption for the recommended minimum duration based on stent type without recurrence of clopidogrel hypersensitivity. There were 59 patients (95%) who had complete resolution of hypersensitivity symptoms at 5±2 days. All but one had treatment in an outpatient setting due to required monitoring in an inpatient setting for angioedema without discontinuation of clopidogrel. A single course of the steroid taper was effective in all but one patient, who required a second course to yield complete resolution of symptoms.

Interestingly, four patients in the study group were re-exposed to clopidogrel and all experienced a recurrence of a clopidogrel hypersensitivity reaction. A repeat course of steroid taper without interruption of clopidogrel therapy proved effective once again. Of note, this is of a similar pattern of a recurrent hypersensitivity reaction as seen with cessation of the medication (as in medication non-compliance) in patients who underwent successful medication desensitization. Therefore, one should be aware that a patient may developed recurrent symptoms of clopidogrel hypersensitivity on subsequent exposures despite a history of successful short course steroid therapy. Accordingly, it may be anticipated that a subsequent treatment course will be required for future exposure to clopidogrel. In addition, a thorough discussion with patients regarding optimal medication adherence is essential in patients who have undergo successful desensitization of clopidogrel hypersensitivity, as to alerting patients that hypersensitivity symptoms may reoccur upon a period of medication non-adherence.

Table 2. Protocol for the management of clopidogrel hypersensitivity without drug interruption at Thomas Jefferson University Hospital

Initial therapy
• Methylprednisolone taper (Medrol Dosepak®, Pfizer, NY, SA)
• Long-acting non-sedating antihistamine: fexofenedine (Allegra® [Sanofi Aventis, Pars, France]) 180mg daily
• Short-acting antihistamine: diphenhydramine (Benadryl® [McNeil, NJ, USA]) 25-50mg every night
Secondary therapy (for symptom relapse)
• Longer course corticosteroids: prednisone 60mg, taper by 10mg every 3 days
• Leukotriene inhibitor: montelukast (Singulair®, Merck) 10mg daily
• Referral to allergist

Our current approach at Thomas Jefferson University Hospital for the management of clopidogrel hypersensitivity is summarized in Table 2. Duration of antihistamine treatment with or without leukotriene inhibitor therapy should be individualized to the patient. If antihistamine is well-tolerated without the occurrence of excessive drowsiness or dry-mouth, therapy can be considered for the duration of the clopidogrel treatment. Some patients and clinicians opt to discontinue antihistamine therapy earlier without the recurrence of hypersensitivity symptoms. The decision to admit a patient for desensitization should be made based on the severity of the patient's hypersensitivity symptoms. This method of desensitization should generally not be used in patients who experience anaphylaxis, exfoliative dermatitis (i.e. Stevens-Johnson syndrome) or toxic epidermal necrolysis, as there are limited treatments for these life-threatening reactions. When severe or recurrent allergic reaction arise allergy consultation would be appropriate.

CONCLUSION

Antiplatelet therapy with clopidogrel is the cornerstone therapy of many cardiovascular conditions. As clopidogrel recently became a generic brand drug in the USA in 2012, its availability will continue to rise. In turn, this would imply a necessary increase in the awareness of clopidogrel hypersensitivity. Diagnosing clopidogrel hypersensitivity can be challenging, as new medications and drug-impregnated polymer stents are frequently introduced during the same admission following a cardiovascular event. Typically, clopidogrel hypersensitivity occurs during the first 2 weeks of clopidogrel initiation, when drug discontinuation carries the greatest risk for stent thrombosis. In most cases, there are no reliable confirmatory diagnostic tests beyond drug re-challenge and close examination of the patient's clinical history and presentation.

In patients receiving clopidogrel in the post-PCI setting, traditional desensitization protocols have been highly successful in enabling resumption of clopidogrel therapy. Treatment of clopidogrel hypersensitivity with corticosteroid taper and antihistamines without temporary drug discontinuation is successful in 85-100% of cases, and appears to be as successful as traditional desensitization. Most patients with life-threatening and severe hypersensitivity syndromes, including anaphylaxis, Stevens-Johnson syndrome and TENS, should not undergo a treatment strategy of desensitization for drug re-challenging as the risk are likely to outweigh the benefits.

As previously discussed, studies on cross-reactivity to prasugrel and ticagrelor have been limited as the major trials excluded patients with a history of hypersensitivity to clopidogrel. Recent literature has demonstrated cross-reactivity to prasugrel in a small fraction of patients known to demonstrate clopidogrel hypersensitivity, and case reports identified the potential role for a safe drug substitution to prasugrel in these instances with several days of steroids overlapping the prasugrel initiation [9, 25, 26, 27]. These new $P2Y_{12}$

inhibitors are more potent and have sufficient clinical evidence that supports specific cardiovascular indications. However, their use is accompanied by a heightened risk for bleeding. The safety and efficacy of these newer agents as substitute therapy in patients with clopidogrel hypersensitivity remains to be determined. The value of cilostazol and novel antiplatelets, such as vorapaxar, in setting of clopidogrel intolerance also needs further evaluation.

In conclusion, in the post-PCI population, treatment of clopidogrel hypersensitivity with corticosteroids and antihistamines without interruption of clopidogrel remains the preferred approach, especially in patients who are not candidates to take more potent and novel antiplatelets. The elimination of the washout period, as in traditional desensitization protocols, avoids the risk of catastrophic stent thrombosis due to early discontinuation of antiplatelet therapy. Successful treatment enables long-term continuation of therapy and is associated with a low risk of adverse cardiovascular events. In parallel, the success of our approach of enabling the development of physiologic tolerance while continuing drug therapy raises the possibility of alternative pathways to drug desensitization. As this technique is proven successful in the management of clopidogrel hypersensitivity, it may be applicable in the future to other drug hypersensitivities where treatment alternatives are limited.

Acknowledgment

We thank Denise Gidaro for assistance in preparing this chapter.

References

[1] IMS health drug distribution data.
[2] Topol, EJ; Schork, NJ. Catapulting clopidogrel pharmacogenomics forward. *Nat Med.*, 2011 Jan, 17(1), 40-1.
[3] Wells, QS; Delaney, JT; Roden, DM. Genetic determinants of response to cardiovascular drugs. *Curr Opin Cardiol.*, 2012 May, 27(3), 253-61.
[4] Levine, GN; Bates, ER; Blankenship, JC; Bailey, SR; Bittl, JA; Cercek, B; Chambers, CE; Ellis, SG; Guyton, RA; Hollenberg, SM; Khot, UN; Lange, RA; Mauri, L; Mehran, R; Moussa, ID; Mukherjee, D; Nallamothu, BK; Ting, HH. American College of Cardiology Foundation; American Heart Association Task Force on Practice

Guidelines; Society for Cardiovascular Angiography and Interventions. 2011 ACCF/AHA/SCAI Guideline for Percutaneous Coronary Intervention. A report of the American College of Cardiology Foundation/American Heart Association Task Force on Practice Guidelines and the Society for Cardiovascular Angiography and Interventions. *J Am Coll Cardiol.*, 2011 Dec 6, 58(24), e44-122.

[5] Clopidogrel (Plavix), package insert. Bristol-Myers Squibb Company & Sanofi Aventis, NJ, USA (2009).

[6] CAPRIE Steering Committee. A randomized, blinded, trial of clopidogrel versus aspirin in patients at risk of ischemic events (CAPRIE). CAPRIE Steering Committee. *Lancet.* 1996 Nov 16, 348(9038), 1329-39.

[7] von Tiehl, KF; Price, MJ; Valencia, R; Ludington, KJ; Teirstein, PS; Simon, RA. Clopidogrel desensitization after drug-eluting stent placement. *J Am Coll Cardiol.*, 2007 Nov 20, 50(21), 2039-43.

[8] Campbell, KL; Cohn, JR; Fischman, DL; Walinsky, P; Mallya, R; Jaffrani, W; Savage, MP. Management of clopidogrel hypersensitivity without drug interruption. *Am J Cardiol.*, 2011 Mar 15, 107(6), 812-6.

[9] Cheema, AN; Mohammad, A; Hong, T; Jakubovic, HR; Parmar, GS; Sharieff, W; Garvey, MB; Kutryk, MJ; Fam, NP; Graham, JJ; Chisholm, RJ. Characterization of clopidogrel hypersensitivity reactions and management with oral steroids without clopidogrel discontinuation. *J Am Coll Cardiol.*, 2011 Sep 27, 58(14), 1445-54.

[10] Palmerini, T; Kirtane, AJ; Serruys, PW; Smits, PC; Kedhi, E; Kereiakes, D; Sangiorgi, D; Bacchi, Reggiani, L; Kaiser, C; Kim, HS; De, Waha, A; Ribichini, F; Stone, GW. Stent thrombosis with everolimus-eluting stents: meta-analysis of comparative randomized controlled trials. Circ Cardiovasc *Interv.*, 2012 Jun, 5(3), 357-64.

[11] van Werkum, JW; Heestermans, AA; Zomer, AC; Kelder, JC; Suttorp, MJ; Rensing, BJ; Koolen, JJ; Brueren, BR; Dambrink, JH; Hautvast, RW; Verheugt, FW; ten, Berg, JM. Predictors of coronary stent thrombosis: the Dutch Stent Thrombosis Registry. *J Am Coll Cardiol.*, 2009 Apr 21, 53(16), 1399-409.

[12] Leon, MB; Baim, DS; Popma, JJ; Gordon, PC; Cutlip, DE; Ho, KK; Giambartolomei, A; Diver, DJ; Lasorda, DM; Williams, DO; Pocock, SJ; Kuntz, RE. A clinical trial comparing three antithrombotic-drug regimens after coronary-artery stenting. Stent Anticoagulation Restenosis Study Investigators. *N Engl J Med.*, 1998 Dec 3, 339(23), 1665-71.

[13] Gent, M; Blakely, JA; Easton, JD; Ellis, DJ; Hachinski, VC; Harbison, JW; Panak, E; Roberts, RS; Sicurella, J; Turpie, AG. The Canadian American Ticlopidine Study (CATS) in thromboembolic stroke. *Lancet.* 1989 Jun 3, 1(8649), 1215-20.

[14] Hass, WK; Easton, JD; Adams, HP, Jr; Pryse-Phillips, W; Molony, BA; Anderson, S; Kamm, B. A randomized trial comparing ticlopidine hydrochloride with aspirin for the prevention of stroke in high-risk patients. Ticlopidine Aspirin Stroke Study Group. *N Engl J Med.*, 1989 Aug 24, 321(8), 501-7.

[15] Biondi-Zoccai, GG; Agostoni, P; Sangiorgi, GM; Iakovou, I; Antoniucci, D; Grube, E; Tamburino, C; Di, Mario, C; Reimers, B; Michev, I; Goktekin, O; Airoldi, F; Chieffo, A; Cosgrave, J; Tassanawiwat, W; Colombo, A. TRUE (Taxus in Real-Life Usage Evaluation) Study Investigators. Comparison of ticlopidine vs. clopidogrel in addition to aspirin after paclitaxel-eluting stent implantation: insights from the TRUE (Taxusin Real-life Usage Evaluation) Study. *Int J Cardiol.*, 2006 Apr 14, 108(3), 406-7.

[16] Ticlopidine hydrochloride, tablet package insert. Genpharm Inc., Toronto, Canada (2002).

[17] Steinhubl, SR; Tan, WA; Foody, JM; Topol, EJ. Incidence and clinical course of thrombotic thrombocytopenic purpura due to ticlopidine following coronary stenting. EPISTENT Investigators. Evaluation of Platelet IIb/IIIa Inhibitor for Stenting. *JAMA.* 1999 Mar 3, 281(9), 806-10.

[18] Walker, NE; Fasano, MB; Horwitz, PA. Desensitization for the management of clopidogrel hypersensitivity: initial clinical experience. *J Invasive Cardiol.*, 2006 Jul, 18(7), 341-4.

[19] Camara, MG; Almeda, FQ. Clopidogrel (Plavix) desensitization: a case series. *Catheter Cardiovasc Interv.*, 2005 Aug, 65(4), 525-7.

[20] Makkar, K; Wilensky, RL; Julien, MB; Herrmann, HC; Spinler, SA. Rash with both clopidogrel and ticlopidine in two patients following percutaneous coronary intervention with drug-eluting stents. *Ann Pharmacother.*, 2006 Jun, 40(6), 1204-7.

[21] Lokhandwala, JO; Best, PJ; Butterfield, JH; Skelding, KA; Scott, T; Blankenship, JC; Buckley, JW; Berger, PB. Frequency of allergic or hematologic adverse reactions to ticlopidine among patients with allergic or hematologic adverse reactions to clopidogrel. *Circ Cardiovasc Interv.*, 2009 Aug, 2(4), 348-51.

[22] Wiviott, SD; Braunwald, E; McCabe, CH; Montalescot, G; Ruzyllo, W; Gottlieb, S; Neumann, FJ; Ardissino, D; De Servi, S; Murphy, SA; Riesmeyer, J; Weerakkody, G; Gibson, CM; Antman, EM. TRITON-TIMI 38 Investigators. Prasugrel versus clopidogrel in patients with acute coronary syndromes. *N Engl J Med.*, 2007 Nov 15, 357(20), 2001-15. Epub, 2007 Nov 4.

[23] Effient (prasugrel), package insert. *Daiichi-Sankyo and Eli Lilly*, IN, USA (2009).

[24] Roe, MT; Armstrong, PW; Fox, KA; White, HD; Prabhakaran, D; Goodman, SG; Cornel, JH; Bhatt, DL; Clemmensen, P; Martinez, F; Ardissino, D; Nicolau, JC; Boden, WE; Gurbel, PA; Ruzyllo, W; Dalby, AJ; McGuire, DK; Leiva-Pons, JL; Parkhomenko, A; Gottlieb, S; Topacio, GO; Hamm, C; Pavlides, G; Goudev, AR; Oto, A; Tseng, CD; Merkely, B; Gasparovic, V; Corbalan, R; Cinteză, M; McLendon, RC; Winters, KJ; Brown, EB; Lokhnygina, Y; Aylward, PE; Huber, K; Hochman, JS; Ohman, EM. TRILOGY ACS Investigators. Prasugrel versus clopidogrel for acute coronary syndromes without revascularization. *N Engl J Med.*, 2012 Oct 4, 367(14), 1297-309.

[25] van Werkum, JW; Braber, TL; Verheggen, PW; Van Der, Have-Roeffel, SM. Prasugrel as alternative treatment strategy in a case with a hypersensitivity reaction to clopidogrel. *Platelets.*, 2011, 22(1), 77-8.

[26] Chopra, P; Verma, P; Klaustermeyer, WB. Successful use of prasugrel, an alternative antiplatelet agent, in a patient with clopidogrel allergy. *Ann Allergy Asthma Immunol.*, 2011 Dec, 107(6), 541-2.

[27] Peppard, SR; Held-Godgluck, BM; Beddingfield, R. Use of prasugrel in a patient with clopidogrel hypersensitivity. *Ann Pharmacother.*, 2011 Oct, 45(10), e54.

[28] Wallentin, L; Becker, RC; Budaj, A; Cannon, CP; Emanuelsson, H; Held, C; Horrow, J; Husted, S; James, S; Katus, H; Mahaffey, KW; Scirica, BM; Skene, A; Steg, PG; Storey, RF; Harrington, RA; PLATO, Investigators; Freij, A; Thorsén, M. Ticagrelor versus clopidogrel in patients with acute coronary syndromes. *N Engl J Med.*, 2009 Sep 10, 361(11), 1045-57. doi: 10.1056/NEJMoa0904327. Epub, 2009 Aug 30.

[29] Wiviott, SD; Antman, EM; Gibson, CM; Montalescot, G; Riesmeyer, J; Weerakkody, G; Winters, KJ; Warmke, JW; McCabe, CH; Braunwald, E. TRITON-TIMI 38 Investigators. Evaluation of prasugrel compared with clopidogrel in patients with acute coronary syndromes: design and rationale for the TRial to assess Improvement in Therapeutic Outcomes by optimizing platelet InhibitioN with prasugrel Thrombolysis In

Myocardial Infarction 38 (TRITON-TIMI 38). *Am Heart J.*, 2006 Oct, 152(4), 627-35.

[30] James, S; Akerblom, A; Cannon, CP; Emanuelsson, H; Husted, S; Katus, H; Skene, A; Steg, PG; Storey, RF; Harrington, R; Becker, R; Wallentin, L. Comparison of ticagrelor, the first reversible oral P2Y(12) receptor antagonist, with clopidogrel in patients with acute coronary syndromes: Rationale, design, and baseline characteristics of the PLATelet inhibition and patient Outcomes (PLATO) trial. *Am Heart J.*, 2009 Apr, 157(4), 599-605.

[31] Bertrand, ME; Legrand, V; Boland, J; Fleck, E; Bonnier, J; Emmanuelson, H; Vrolix, M; Missault, L; Chierchia, S; Casaccia, M; Niccoli, L; Oto, A; White, C; Webb-Peploe, M; Van, Belle, E; McFadden, EP. Randomized multicenter comparison of conventional anticoagulation versus antiplatelet therapy in unplanned and elective coronary stenting. The full anticoagulation versus aspirin and ticlopidine (fantastic) study. *Circulation.*, 1998 Oct 20, 98(16), 1597-603.

[32] Schömig, A; Neumann, FJ; Kastrati, A; Schühlen, H; Blasini, R; Hadamitzky, M; Walter, H; Zitzmann-Roth, EM; Richardt, G; Alt, E; Schmitt, C; Ulm, K. A randomized comparison of antiplatelet and anticoagulant therapy after the placement of coronary-artery stents. *N Engl J Med.*, 1996 Apr 25, 334(17), 1084-9.

[33] Ge, J; Han, Y; Jiang, H; Sun, B; Chen, J; Zhang, S; Du, Z. RACTS (Randomized Prospective Antiplatelet Trial of Cilostazol Versus Ticlopidine in Patients Undergoing Coronary Stenting) Trial Investigators. RACTS: a prospective randomized antiplatelet trial of cilostazol versus ticlopidine in patients undergoing coronary stenting: long-term clinical and angiographic outcome. *J Cardiovasc Pharmacol.*, 2005 Aug, 46(2), 162-6.

[34] Lee, SW; Park, SW; Hong, MK; Lee, CW; Kim, YH; Park, JH; Kang, SJ; Han, KH; Kim, JJ; Park, SJ. Comparison of cilostazol and clopidogrel after successful coronary stenting. *Am J Cardiol.*, 2005 Apr 1, 95(7), 859-62.

[35] Park, SJ; Shim, WH; Ho, DS; Raizner, AE; Park, SW; Hong, MK; Lee, CW; Choi, D; Jang, Y; Lam, R; Weissman, NJ; Mintz, GS. A paclitaxel-eluting stent for the prevention of coronary restenosis. *N Engl J Med.*, 2003 Apr 17, 348(16), 1537-45.

[36] Ahn, Y; Jeong, MH; Jeong, JW; Kim, KH; Ahn, TH; Kang, WC; Park, CG; Kim, JH; Chae, IH; Nam, CW; Hur, SH; Bae, JH; Kim, KY; Oh, SK. Randomized comparison of cilostazol vs clopidogrel after drug-

eluting stenting in diabetic patients--cilostazol for diabetic patients in drug-eluting stent (CIDES) trial. *Circ J.*, 2008 Jan, 72(1), 35-9.

[37] Guyatt, GH; Akl, EA; Crowther, M; Gutterman, DD; Schuünemann, HJ. American College of Chest Physicians Antithrombotic Therapy and Prevention of Thrombosis Panel. Executive summary: Antithrombotic Therapy and Prevention of Thrombosis, 9th ed: American College of Chest Physicians Evidence-Based Clinical Practice Guidelines. *Chest.*, 2012 Feb, 141(2 Suppl), 7S-47S.

[38] Packer, M; Carver, JR; Rodeheffer, RJ; Ivanhoe, RJ; DiBianco, R; Zeldis, SM; Hendrix, GH; Bommer, WJ; Elkayam, U; Kukin, ML, et al. Effect of oral milrinone on mortality in severe chronic heart failure. The PROMISE Study Research Group. *N Engl J Med.*, 1991 Nov 21, 325(21), 1468-75.

[39] Pletal (cilostazol), package insert. Otsuka America Pharmaceutical, MD, USA (1999).

[40] Tricoci, P; Huang, Z; Held, C; Moliterno, DJ; Armstrong, PW; Van, de, Werf, F; White, HD; Aylward, PE; Wallentin, L; Chen, E; Lokhnygina, Y; Pei, J; Leonardi, S; Rorick, TL; Kilian, AM; Jennings, LH; Ambrosio, G; Bode, C; Cequier, A; Cornel, JH; Diaz, R; Erkan, A; Huber, K; Hudson, MP; Jiang, L; Jukema, JW; Lewis, BS; Lincoff, AM; Montalescot, G; Nicolau, JC; Ogawa, H; Pfisterer, M; Prieto, JC; Ruzyllo, W; Sinnaeve, PR; Storey, RF; Valgimigli, M; Whellan, DJ; Widimsky, P; Strony, J; Harrington, RA; Mahaffey, KW. TRACER Investigators. Thrombin-receptor antagonist vorapaxar in acute coronary syndromes. *N Engl J Med.*, 2012 Jan 5, 366(1), 20-33.

[41] Morrow, DA; Braunwald, E; Bonaca, MP; Ameriso, SF; Dalby, AJ; Fish, MP; Fox, KA; Lipka, LJ; Liu, X; Nicolau, JC; Ophuis, AJ; Paolasso, E; Scirica, BM; Spinar, J; Theroux, P; Wiviott, SD; Strony, J; Murphy, SA. TRA 2P–TIMI 50 Steering Committee and Investigators. Vorapaxar in the secondary prevention of atherothrombotic events. *N Engl J Med.*, 2012 Apr 12, 366(15), 1404-13.

[42] Solensky, R. Drug desensitization. *Immunol Allergy Clin North Am.*, 2004 Aug,24(3), 425-43, vi.

[43] de Groot, H; Mulder, WM; Terreehorst, I. Utility of desensitization for allergy to antibiotics. *Neth J Med.*, 2012 Mar, 70(2), 58-62.

[44] Stevenson, DD. Aspirin sensitivity and desensitization for asthma and sinusitis. *Curr Allergy Asthma Rep.*, 2009 Mar, 9(2), 155-63.

[45] Solensky, R. Drug hypersensitivity. Med. *Clin. North Am.*, 90, 233-260 (2006).

[46] Miller, MM; Miller, MM. Beta-blockers and anaphylaxis: are the risks overstated? *J Allergy Clin Immunol.*, 2005 Oct,116(4), 931-3. author reply 933-6.

[47] Vigo, PG; MacDowell, AL; Wedner, HJ. Successful desensitization with clopidogrel after a positive skin test. *Ann Allergy Asthma Immunol*, 2005, 94, 132.

[48] Camara, MG; Almeda, FQ. Clopidogrel (Plavix) desensitization: a case series. *Catheter Cardiovasc Interv.*, 2005 August, 65(4), 525-7.

[49] Lee-Wong, M; Gadhvi, D; Resnick, D. Clopidogrel desensitization. *Ann Allergy Asthma Immunol.*, 2006 May, 96(5), 756-7.

[50] Walker, NE; Fasano, MB; Hobbs, RA; Horwitz, PA. Clopidogrel desensitization protocol for the treatment of thienopyridine hypersensitivity. *Crit Pathw Cardiol.*, 2007 Mar, 6(1), 26-9.

[51] Owen, P; Garner, J; Hergott, L; Page, RL, 2nd. Clopidogrel desensitization: case report and review of published protocols. *Pharmacotherapy.*, 2008 Feb, 28(2), 259-70.

[52] Kammer, RT. Successful clopidogrel desensitization after drug-eluting stent implantation. *J Invasive Cardiol.*, 2009 Mar, 21(3), 134-5.

[53] Campbell, KL; Cohn, JR; Savage, MP. Clopidogrel hypersensitivity: clinical challenges and options for management. *Expert Rev Clin Pharmacol.*, 2010 Jul, 3(4), 553-61.

In: Clopidogrel
Editors: J. P. Alesci and A. Victorino
ISBN: 978-1-62948-336-8
© 2014 Nova Science Publishers, Inc.

Chapter 6

CLOPIDOGREL AND GASTROINTESTINAL HARM

Parth J. Parekh[1], Edward C. Oldfield IV [2*] and David A. Johnson[3]
[1]Department of Internal Medicine, Eastern Virginia Medical School, Norfolk, VA, US
[2]MD Candidate 2015, Eastern Virginia Medical School University School, Norfolk, VA, US
[3]Department of Internal Medicine, Division of Gastroenterology, Eastern Virginia Medical School, Norfolk, VA, US

ABSTRACT

Proton pump inhibitors often are prescribed in combination with clopidogrel to decrease the risk of gastrointestinal bleeding after an acute coronary syndrome. Clopidogrel is a prodrug that has to be metabolized in the liver to generate the active metabolite. Both medications are metabolized largely by the CYP2C19 enzyme, therefore concerns exist that a drug–drug interaction during concomitant treatment may result in a reduction of platelet inhibition. We have reviewed the observational and randomized control studies that have evaluated the potential influence of proton pump inhibitors on the inhibitory effect of clopidogrel, along with cardiovascular outcomes. We summarized regulatory and academic

* Corresponding author: ecoldfield@gmail.com.

guidelines for treatment of patients in which concomitant therapy with clopidogrel and proton pump inhibitors may be indicated. Lastly we discuss confounding issues such as the differential effects of individual proton pump inhibitors on the pharmacodynamics of clopidogrel and variation in clopidogrel metabolism mediated by genetic polymorphisms of the CYP2C19 isoenzyme.

I. INTRODUCTION

Each year in the United States 635,000 Americans suffer from an acute myocardial infarction(MI) resulting in over 954,000 percutaneous coronary interventions(PCI).[1] For many of these patients a common mainstay of treatment is dual-antiplatelet therapy with aspirin(ASA) and a $P2Y_{12}$ inhibitor. Clopidogrel is the most commonly prescribed $P2Y_{12}$ inhibitor and is available as a low-cost generic.[2,3] Clopidogrel (Plavix®) is a thienopyridine antiplatelet agent that is approved for use in individuals with acute coronary syndrome(ACS) (non-ST-segment elevation myocardial infarction(NSTEMI), unstable angina, ST-segment elevation myocardial infarction(STEMI)) who are to be either managed medically or with coronary revascularization. In addition, clopidogrel is also indicated for use in individuals who have suffered a recent MI , stroke or have established peripheral arterial disease to reduce the risk of ischemic stroke, new MI or other vascular death.[4]

With such a large number of individuals taking clopidogrel it is essential that physicians understand the potential for adverse events, in particular gastrointestinal (GI) harm. Dual-antiplatelet therapy has been postulated to cause direct GI injury, but more importantly it has been shown to have the potential for exacerbation of pre-existing GI injury from non-steroidal anti-inflammatory drugs (NSAIDs) or *H. pylori*.[5] As such proton pump inhibitors (PPIs) are recommended treatment for any individual with a previous history or multiple risk factors for an upper GI bleed. Risk factors include advanced age, use of anticoagulants, steroids, NSAIDs, or *H. pylori* infection.[6]

Recently, much controversy has developed around the co-administration of clopidogrel with PPIs. This first began in January 2009 when the Food and Drug Administration (FDA) issued a recommendation against the combined use of clopidogrel and all PPIs. The FDA subsequently revised their statement to recommend against concomitant use of clopidorel with potent CYP2C19 inhibitors, namely omeprazole, esomeprazole, and the H2 receptor antagonist cimetidine.[7,8] Since then, this has become an area of intense focus with numerous studies offering conflicting viewpoints. This chapter aims to outline the risks associated with clopidogrel and adverse GI events, explore the pharmacokinetic and pharmacodynamic interactions between clopidogrel and PPIs, outline the treatment strategies, discuss clinical significance and offer guidance.

II. Clopidogrel and GI Harm

Mechanism of Clopidogrel-Associated GI Harm

Normal healing of gastric ulcers relies on the process of platelet aggregation. This results in the release of pro-angiogenic growth factors from platelet α-granules, namely vascular endothelial growth factor (VEGF).[9] Also involved in this process is the anti-angiogenic growth factor, endostatin. Endostatin, while not a component of the platelet granules, appears to be an important mediator of the healing process.. Variations in the ratio of pro-angiogenic to anti-angiogenic factors allow for an ideal environment for proper healing. This has been experimentally documented through the induction of gastric ulcers in a rat model, which showed that mucosal injury led to an increase in VEGF and a decrease in endostatin, necessary for the subsequent steps of mucosal regeneration.[10] Further, inhibition of platelet aggregation through the administration of ticlopidine, a thienopyridine similar to clopidogrel, abolished these normal physiologic shifts in the rat model. Similarly, through this mechanism clopidogrel can aggravate preexisting mucosal irritation from esophagitis, peptic ulcer disease related to *H. pylori*, aspirin and NSAIDs.[11]

Clopidogrel and Upper GI Bleeding

Thienopyridines have been widely shown to significantly reduce the number of major adverse cardiac events (MACE) including cardiac death, MI, stroke. Unfortunately, they simultaneously increase the risk for major bleeding events. Some of the first evidence of this association came from a randomized, double-blind, placebo controlled trial comparing ASA alone to clopidogrel plus ASA. The study found that for patients with a NSTEMI, use of clopidogrel plus ASA showed a reduction in MACE from 11.4% to 9.3% (RR 0.80, 95% CI 0.72-0.90, p= <0.001), but also increased major bleeding events from 2.7% to 3.7% (RR 1.37, p=0.001).[12] Similar findings were reported in another randomized, double-blind study of patients with atrial fibrillation unsuitable for a vitamin K antagonist and met at least one risk criteria for stroke. This study found that the use of clopidogrel plus ASA decreased major vascular events from 7.6% to 6.8%, but major bleeding occurred in 2.0% vs. 1.3% (RR 1.57, 95% CI 129-1.92; p<0.001), respectively.[13] In addition, a secondary analysis of the VALIANT trial (VALsartan In Acute myocardial INfarcTion) consisting of 14,703 high-risk MI survivors, as defined by left ventricular dysfunction and/or heart failure, showed that the dual-antiplatelet therapy was the most significant predictor for GI bleeding (HR 3.18, 95% CI 1.91-5.29).[14] Most recently, a cohort study with nested case-controlled analysis of 20,000 patients from The Health Improvement Network (THIN) in the UK, reviewed the relative risk of various medications and their impact on upper GI bleeding (UGIB).[15] The analysis revealed clopidogrel alone was associated with an increased risk for UGIB (RR 1.67, 95% CI 1.24-2.24) and that co-adminsitration of clopidogrel and ASA presented an increased risk over ASA alone (RR 2.08, 95% CI 1.34-3.21).[15]

Clopidogrel and Lower GI Bleeding

While the relationship between antiplatelet and PPI co-therapy with UGIB is quite evident, recent evidence suggests more attention should be paid to lower GI bleeds. An observational study with prospective follow up for 1,219 patients undergoing PCI found that lower GI bleeding occurred more frequently than UGIB at 74% versus 26%, respectively. [16] Importantly, of the 27 patients that developed a GI bleed, 25 were on dual-antiplatelet therapy at the time. The authors attributed the increased frequency of GI bleeding to antiplatelet therapy unmasking previously existing lesions. Despite the large number of bleeds related to dual-antiplatelet therapy, the authors found that in a multivariate analysis the only risk factors for predicting GI bleeding were a history of peptic ulcer disease and warfarin treatment, not dual-antiplatelet therapy.

ACCF/ACG/AHA Expert Consensus Guidelines [17]

This expert consensus document was developed by the American College of Cardiology Foundation (ACCF), the American College of Gastroenterology

(ACG), and the American Heart Association (AHA) to review the recent developments in this area, provide guidance for clinical management and highlight areas of future research necessary to address current knowledge gaps. As a result of the increased risk for UGIB, this consensus document suggests the co-administration of a PPI for any individual on dual anti-platelet therapy at high risk for UGIB. Additionally, several topics pertaining clopidogrel and its interaction with PPIs were addressed in this consensus.

The two main hypotheses regarding the interaction between clopidogrel and PPIs center on the CYP450 enzyme pathway, namely CYP2C19. The first hypothesis described the reduced action of clopidogrel through competitive metabolic effects. It stated that concomitant use of PPIs might affect CYP2C19, which isrequired for metabolizing clopidogrel to its active form, thus decreasing its antiplatelet effect. Pharmacokinetic studies in vitro suggest that all PPIs inhibit CYP2C19 to some extent however, the strongest evidence for an interaction is between omeprazole and clopidogrel.

The second hypothesis described the genetic polymorphisms and its role in the metabolism of clopidogrel from its prodrug form to an active metabolite. Those who are genetically poor metabolizers may be more susceptible to cardiovascular events as a result of reduced platelet inhibition. Later sections in this chapter will contain a more in depth analysis of the various alleles that dictate the metabolic activity of the CYP2C19 isoenzyme.

PPIs, a Mechanism for Improved Adherence?

In addition to the decreased risk for GI bleeding, PPI administration may also be associated with improved adherence to dual-antiplatelet therapy.[18] A recent cohort study assessing the risk for discontinuation of dual-antiplatelet therapy after placement of a drug eluding stent demonstrated that failure of adherence led to an increase in the hazard ratio for stent thrombosis to 89.78 (95% CI 29.90-269.60).[19] The addition of a PPI to the treatment regimen has also been noted in an ongoing phase III trial of PA32540, a 325 mg enteric coated aspirin plus 40mg of immediate release omeprazole. PA32540 in comparison to 325mg of enteric coated aspirin alone revealed a significant increase in adherence at 6 months.[20] Within the study group, discontinuation of medication due to upper GI adverse events was 1.5% in the PA32540 group versus 8.2% in the aspirin group and discontinuation due to any adverse event was 6.7% in the PA32540 group versus 11.2% in the aspirin group.[19] Even though this study did not include clopidogrel, it highlights the potential benefit of PPIs in improving adherence along with a decreased risk for GI bleeding.

III. Clopidogrel and Proton Pump Inhibitor Interactions

Pharmacodynamics

Clopidogrel is a prodrug, which when metabolized into its active compound irreversibly binds to the $P2Y_{12}$ receptor. This inhibits ADP-mediated platelet activation of the glycoprotein IIb/IIIa complex and subsequent platelet aggregation.[21] Approximately 15% of absorbed clopidogrel is converted into the active metabolite responsible for inhibition of platelet aggregation.[22] The CYP2C19 and CYP3A4 enzymes primarily mediate the conversion of clopidogrel from the prodrug form to its active metabolite.[23] The reliance on the 2C19 and 3A4 cytochrome enzymes, common sites of inhibition for several PPIs, represents the genesis of the controversy over the potential for clinically significant pharmacokinetic interactions between clopidogrel and PPIs. This process, along with the relevant mediators, is outlined figure 1 below.[24]

Another site of potential drug interaction with clopidogrel is through the P-glycoprotein intestinal efflux transporter, also known as MDR1 (multidrug resistance transporter 1) or ABCB1 (ATP-binding cassette, subfamily B (MDR), member 1). The P-glycoprotein intestinal efflux transporter is responsible for transporting drugs from the enterocyte into the intestinal lumen for excretion.[25] Proton pump inhibitors are both substrates and inhibitors of P-glycoprotein and as such have the capacity to alter clopidogrel absorption.[26] In theory alteration of P-glycoprotein function from either induction, inhibition, or reduced function from altered genetic alleles, has the potential to cause further pharmacokinetic interactions with CYP450 enzymes and ultimately clopidogrel absorption and metabolism. Currently, there is insufficient data for any clinical application, however the uncertain potential of PPI interactions with the intestinal absorption of clopidogrel through the P-glycoprotein mechanism may be a focus of future research.

Pharmacokinetics: Measuring Clopidogrel Activity

As previously discussed, the clopidogrel irreversibly binds to the $P2Y_{12}$ receptor on platelets thus inhibiting the process of platelet aggregation. While numerous platelet aggregation tests exist, current studies have primarily relied on two tests for determination of clopidogrel activity. Vasodilator-stimulated phosphoprotein (VASP) is a cytoskeleton-associated protein whose phosphorylation correlates with the level of glycoprotein IIb/IIIa inhibition.[27] In this manner, the use of a Platelet Reactivity Index (PRI) serves as a selective indicator for the metabolic activity of clopidogrel by measuring the level of VASP phosphorylation. Current testing for individual responses to clopidogrel via the PRI has led to the development of a simple classification of good responders versus poor responders based on a PRI of less than 50% for good responders or greater than 50% for poor responders.[28] This is in contrast to the previous standard for assessing clopidogrel activity, which involved light transmission aggregometry to determine the percentage of platelet aggregation before and after administration of clopidogrel. Since this method measured platelet aggregation alone, it was not able to selectively discriminate clopidogrel activity from other antiplatelet agents, namely ASA.[29]

CYP Allele Status: Genetic Polymorphisms for Drug Metabolism

One of the most recent advances in estimating clopidogrel response comes from the ability to genotype CYP2C19 allele status. While there are 3 alleles associated with decreased metabolism, CYP2C19*2, *3, *4, it is primarily CYP2C19*2 that is best characterized with the prevalence of this allele estimated at 30% of whites, 40% of blacks, and 55% of East Asians.[30] The decreased metabolism from the reduced function alleles results in less conversion from the prodrug form to its active metabolite, hence a net decrease in clopidogrel effectiveness. A study of healthy volunteers with this reduced function allele showed decreased exposure to the active metabolite of clopidogrel by 32.4% compared to non-carriers and also an absolute reduction in maximal platelet aggregation by 9%.[31] Importantly, this association has not been documented with prasugrel, an alternative thienopyridine to clopidogrel.[32]

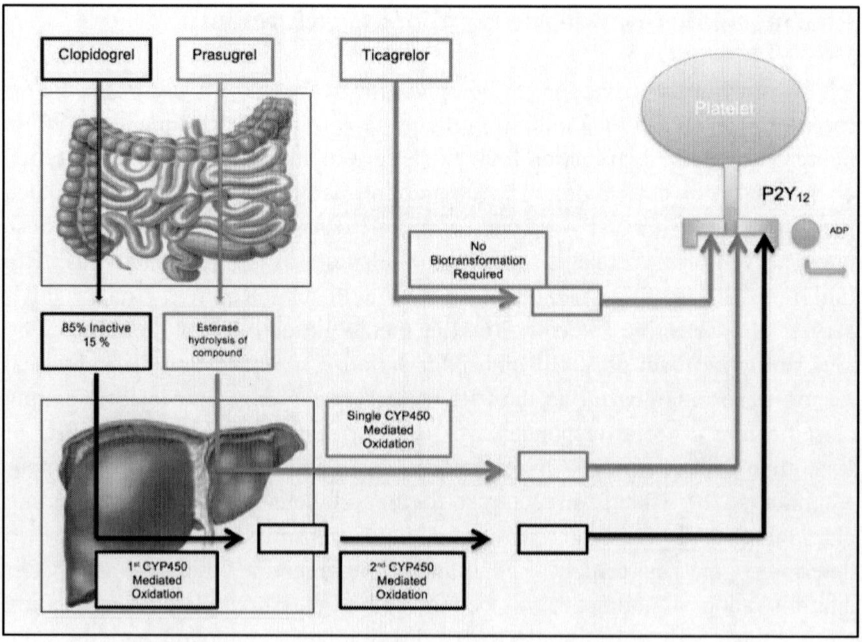

Figure 1. Current FDA Labeling for PPIs.

Despite well documented evidence for reduced function in platelet studies, the clinical significance of the CYP2C19*2 allele is not as well defined. In a recent prospective study, the allele status and concurrent use of PPIs or calcium channel blockers (CCB) were collected from 1,069 patients undergoing PCI for coronary artery disease. Results showed that patients with an allele associated with decreased clopidogrel metabolism are not at an increased risk for adverse cardiovascular events. Additionally, PPI use in combination with such an allele was not associated with increased risk; rather, PPI use was only associated with increased cardiovascular risk for individuals with reduced function alleles also on a CCB (HR 3.3, 95% CI 1.0-5.3, p=0.044).[33] By comparison, a clinically significant finding was noted during a side-by-side analysis of clopidogrel and prasugrel in the TRITON-TIMI trial, in which 2,932 patients with ACS were genotyped for both the CYP2C19 allele and ABC1B1 C3435T status (decreased expression of the gene encoding P-glycoprotein) and placed on either clopidogrel or prasugrel.[34] Subgroup analysis of the clopidogrel arm revealed that ABCIB1 C3435T increased cardiovascular risk both independently and in complement to CYP2C19 reduced function allele, while there was no significant interaction or increased risk in the prasugrel arm.

Currently, conflicting information on the clinical significance of genetic polymorphisms for CYP2C19 and P-glycoprotein prevents a strict determination of an absolute risk; however, as more information becomes available, this will certainly become a focal point of future research. Given the decreasing cost of genotyping, these polymorphisms have the potential to become a mainstay of clinical practice and allow optimal tailoring of treatment regimens based on individual risk. As such, clinicians should be aware of these polymorphisms and their potential for clinically significant interactions.

This section will cover the reported evidence for an interaction with clopidogrel, if any, directly from the manufacturers information. All data in this section is taken from the current FDA product information and labeling for each of the drugs. Subsequently, we will cover the current literature available on the reported variations among PPIs as they relate to pharmacokinetic interactions with clopidogrel in the next section.

Omeprazole (Prilosec®, Prilosec OTC®, Zegerid®)[35]

In a crossover study, 72 healthy subjects were administered clopidogrel (300 mg loading dose followed by 75 mg per day maintenance dose) alone and with concomitant use with omeprazole (80 mg at the same time as clopidogrel) for 5 days duration. When administered together, the exposure to the active metabolite of clopidogrel was decreased by 46% on day 1 and 42% by day 5. A second crossover study showed a similar pharmacokinetic interaction when clopidogrel (300 mg loading dose following by a maintenance dose of 75 mg daily) and omeprazole 80 mg were co-administered for 30 days with exposure to the active metabolite as being reduced by 41% to 46% over this time period.

Current manufacturer recommendations are to avoid concomitant use of omeprazole with clopidogrel given the impaired metabolism of clopidogrel into its active metabolite from the direct effect of omeprazole on CYP2C19 activity.

Esomeprazole (Nexium®)[36]

Results from a cross over study in which healthy subjects were co-administered clopidogrel (300 mg loading dose followed by 75 mg per day maintenance dose) and esomeprazole (40 mg daily) for 30 days demonstrated a 35% to 40% reduction in the exposure to the active metabolite of clopidogrel.

Current manufacturer recommendations are to avoid concomitant use of esomeprazole with clopidogrel given the impaired metabolism of clopidogrel into its active metabolite from the direct effect of esomeprazole on CYP2C19 activity.

Lansoprazole (Prevacid®)[37]

A study of 40 healthy subjects who were CYP2C19 extensive metabolizers were administered clopidogrel 75 mg alone or concomitantly with lansoprazole 30 mg for 9 days. The mean area under the curve (AUC) of the active metabolite of clopidogrel was reduced by approximately 14% (mean AUC ratio was 86%, with 90% CI of 80 to 92%) when lansoprazole was co-administered with clopidogrel as compared to administration of clopidogrel alone. The pharmacokinetic interaction was also measured demonstrating a change in the inhibition of platelet aggregation (induced by 5 *u*mol ADP) that was related to the change in exposure to the active metabolite of clopidogrel, however, the clinical significance of this finding is not clear.

Current manufacturer recommendations do not require any dose adjustment of clopidogrel with co-administration of an approved dose of lansoprazole.

Dexlansoprazole (Dexilant®)[38]

A study of 40 healthy subjects who were CYP2C19 extensive metabolizers were administered clopidogrel 75 mg alone or concomitantly with dexlansoprazole 60 mg for a duration of 9 days. The mean AUC of the active metabolite of clopidogrel was reduced by approximately 9% (mean AUC ratio was 91%, with 90% CI of 86-97%) when dexlansoprazole was co-administered with clopidogrel as compared to the administration of clopidogrel alone. The pharmacokinetic interaction was also measured demonstrating a change in the inhibition of platelet aggregation (induced by 5 *u*mol ADP) that was related to the change in exposure to the active metabolite of clopidogrel, however, the clinical significance of this finding is not clear.

Current manufacturer recommendations do not require any dose adjustment of clopidogrel with co-administration of an approved dose of dexlansoprazole.

Pantoprazole (Protonix®)[39]

A crossover study of 66 healthy subjects who were administered either clopidogrel alone (300 mg loading dose followed by a 75 mg per day maintenance dose) or concomitantly with pantoprazole (80 mg per day) for duration of 5 days. Results of the study demonstrated that on day 5 the mean AUC of the active metabolite of clopidogrel was reduced by approximately 14% (geometric mean ratio was 86%, with 90% CI of 79 to 93%) when pantoprazole was co-administered with clopidogrel as compared to clopidogrel administered alone. The pharmacokinetic interaction was also measured demonstrating a change in the inhibition of platelet aggregation (induced by 5 *u*mol ADP) that was related to the change in exposure to the active metabolite of clopidogrel, however, the clinical significance of this finding is not clear. [39]

A recent randomized controlled trial has suggested that there is a significant interference of clopidogrel antiplatelet effect when concomitantly administered with pantoprazole. Parri et al. randomized 105 patients with STEMI undergoing PCI also receiving dual antiplatelet therapy to pantoprazole (n=54) or ranitidine (n=51).[40] Residual platelet reactivity was then evaluated by ways of Platelet Function Analyzer-100 and by light transmitted aggregometry with 10 *u*mol ADP and 1 mM arachidonic acid on days 5 and 30 after PCI. The results showed a significant increase in maximum aggregation with ADP in the patients randomized to pantoprazole at day 5 (p=0.01) and day 30 (p=0.03) which is illustrated below.

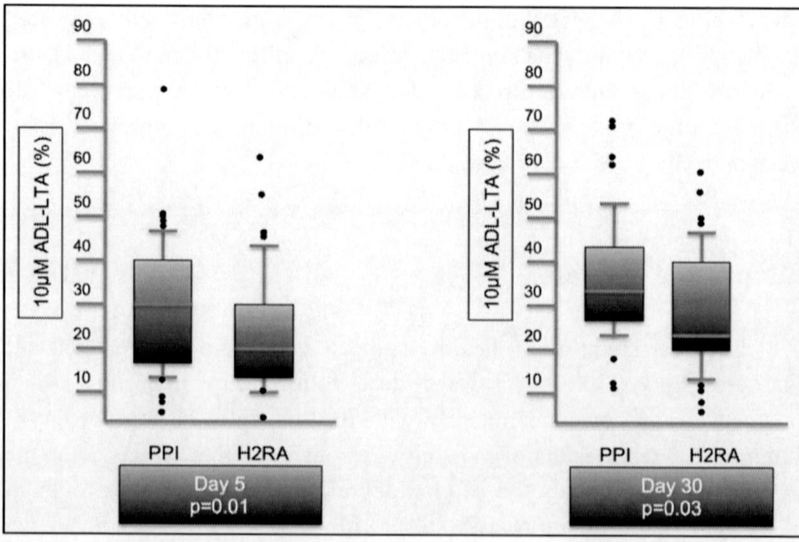

Figure 2. The results showed a significant increase in maximum aggregation with ADP in the patients randomized to pantoprazole at day 5 (p=0.01) and day 30 (p=0.03)

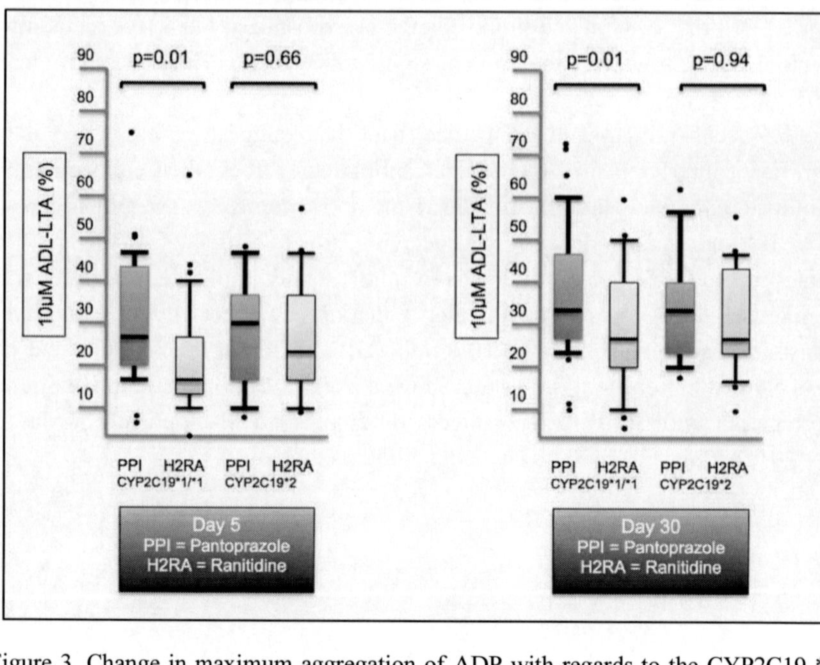

Figure 3. Change in maximum aggregation of ADP with regards to the CYP2C19 *1 and *2 polymorphisms at days 5 and 30 after PCI, respectively. [40]

Albeit a higher prevalence of the CYP2C19*2 allele in the ranitdine group (40% versus 28% in the PPI group, however, not statistically significant) the sub-analysis demonstrated that the phenotypical data of the platelet function test cannot be analyzed separately from genetic data. The two figures above represent the change in maximum aggregation of ADP with regards to the CYP2C19 *1 and *2 polymorphisms at days 5 and 30 after PCI, respectively. [40].

The authors were able to conclude after regression analysis and correction for the bias of CYP2C19*2 that pantoprazole does increase the maximum aggregation with ADP in patients treated with dual-antiplatelet therapy.[40].

Current manufacturer recommendations do not require any dose adjustment of clopidogrel with co-administration of an approved dose of pantoprazole[39], although the most recent report[40] may raise some new concerns about concomitant dosing.

V. Pharmacokinetic and Pharmacodynamic Evidence for a Clopidogrel-PPI Interaction

Evidence from Platelet Aggregation Studies

Evaluation of platelet aggregation studies to date has revealed conflicting results with substantial variation also reported for intra-class differences among PPIs. Gilard et al evaluated the impact of omeprazole on clopidogrel activity in a randomized, double-blind study of patients undergoing coronary artery stent implantation (n=124).[41] These patients on dual-antiplatelet therapy, with ASA and clopidogrel, were assigned to either omeprazole (20 mg per day) or placebo. Clopidogrel activity was then monitored with PRIs measured at days 1 and 7. After 7 days of treatment, PRIs in the omeprazole group were 51.4% versus 39.8% in the placebo group, indicating a significant decrease in the inhibitory activity of clopidogrel ($p < 0.0001$). Similarly, a post-hoc analysis of the PRINCIPLE-TIMI 44 trial (Prasugrel In Comparison to Clopidogrel for Inhibition of Platelet Activation and Aggregation), which was a randomized, double-blind study of 201 patients undergoing PCI. The results of the study which randomized patients to receive either clopidogrel or prasugrel revealed a significant decrease in platelet inhibition as measured by aggregometry for patients taking both PPIs and clopidogrel.[42] At 24 hours after a loading dose of clopidogrel (600 mg), mean platelet inhibition was decreased with measured inhibition of 50.0% in PPI users versus 18.2% in non-PPI users (p= 0.009). Further, after 15 days of follow up PPI users showed greater than a 6 fold difference in levels of platelet inhibition as compared to non-PPI users (50.0% vs. 7.9%, p=0.012). Importantly, this data came from a post-hoc analysis of PRINICPLE-TIMI trial, which was not designed with randomization of PPI use. As such potential cofounders may exist in particular with the small sample size.

Evidence for Differences between PPIs

Given the FDA recommendation against the use of clopidogrelwith the strong CYP2C19 inhibitors, namely omeprazole and esomeprazole, more research has been dedicated towards outlining the pharmacokinetic interaction between various PPIs. Frelinger et al evaluated the effects of dexlansoprazole, lansoprazole, esomeprazole, and omeprazole on the pharmacokinetic interactions with clopidogrel.[43] This randomized, 2-period, crossover study of 160 healthy subjects, all homozygous CYP2C19 extensive metabolizers, found that omeprazole and esomeprazole, but not dexlansoprazole or lansoprazole, significantly reduced the effects of clopidogrel as measured by the VASP PRI. Further supporting this claim, evidence from the SPICE trial (evaluation of the influence of Statins and Proton pump Inhibitors on Clopidogrel antiplatelet Effects) assessed PRI levels in 277 patients randomized to either rosuvastatin or atorvastatin and then randomized to one of four gastroprotective agents, esomeprazole, omeprazole, pantoprazole, or ranitidine.[44] Among the four agents, only esomeprazole (OR 8.8, 95% CI 3.3-24.9; $p < 0.0001$) and omeprazole (OR 3.0, 95% CI 1.2-8.1; p =0.02) were associated with a change in the PRI of greater than 10%. While pantoprazole was not addressed in this study, Parri et al recently focused on the interaction between pantoprazole and clopidogrel interaction in a prospective randomized control trial of 105 consecutive patients undergoing PCI on dual-antiplatelet therapy assigned to either pantoprazole or ranitidine. This study found that pantoprazole was significantly associated with a greater decrease in clopidogrel activity than ranitidine, as measured by an increase in the maximal aggregation of ADP (p = 0.03). Importantly, a significant difference was only noted for patients carrying the CYP2C19*1 wild type allele, not for those patients with the reduced function CYP2C19*2 allele.

In contrast to the significant finding for PPI interactions, Siller-Matua et al assigned patients undergoing PCI (n=300) to either clopidogrel alone, clopidogrel and esomeprazole, or clopidogrel and pantoprazole.[45] Their findings suggest that neither esomeprazole nor pantoprazole significantly interfered with the metabolic activity of clopidogrel, as measured by both VASP PRI and ADP-induced platelet aggregation.[45] Tunggal et al also reported no significant reduction in the platelet inhibitory effect of clopidogrel for patients randomized to either esomeprazole or the H2 Receptor Antagonist, famotidine.[46] These findings highlight an important point that while famotidine has minimal reported interaction with CYP450 enzymes, it was not significantly different from esomeprazole, which has documented CYP2C19 and 3A4 interactions.[47] These esomeprazole findings were also supported by another recent study of 108 healthy volunteers, assessing the maximum inhibition of platelet aggregation and change in PRI between omeprazole, esomeprazole, and lansoprazole.[48] The results revealed that all three PPIs decreased the antiplatelet effect of clopidogrel and decreased systemic exposure to the active metabolite, however when esomeprazole was administered in combination with dual-antiplatelet therapy (versus clopidogrel alone) no difference in platelet aggregation was found, despite the decreased levels of active metabolite.[48]

Evidence from Clinical Trials

COGENT: Clopidogrel and the Optimization of Gastrointestinal Events Trial

Some of the most convincing evidence against the purported interaction between PPIs and clopidogrel comes from a double-blind, placebo controlled, randomized trial comparing rates of adverse GI and cardiovascular events in patients on clopidogrel with and without omeprazole.[49] At 180 days, adverse GI events were decreased in the omeprazole group at 1.1% versus 2.9% with the placebo group (HR .34 95% CI 0.18-0.63). Additionally, there was no significant difference in adverse cardiovascular events with rates of 4.9% in the omeprazole group versus 5.7% in the placebo group (HR 0.99; 95% CI 0.68-1.44; $p = 0.96$). The results of this randomized trial suggest that in contrast to laboratory studies, which suggest that there are significant drug interactions, in the clinical setting such significance is not apparent at present. Further, the use of omeprazole as the PPI in this study strengthens the outcomes, as omeprazole represents not only the most commonly prescribed PPI in the United States[50], but has also been widely documented as the one of strongest CYP2C19 inhibitor amongst PPIs and therefore more likely to induce clinically significant drug interactions with clopidogrel.[51]

CREDO: Clopidogrel for the Reduction of Events During Obstruction

Dunn et al performed a post-hoc analysis of the CREDO trial evaluating the influence of PPIs on the outcomes of patients randomized to either clopidogrel or placebo who underwent PCI. Their findings revealed that clopidogrel reduced adverse cardiovascular events to a similar degree whether or not a patient was on a PPI, but more importantly that PPI use was independently associated with an increased risk for cardiovascular events at 28 days (HR 1.6, 95% CI 1.08-2.5, p= 0.022) and 1 year (HR 1.5, 95% CI 1.1-2.1, p= 0.012).[52] This finding is in accordance with other studies, which have found PPI use may be a marker for, rather than a cause of, higher rates of adverse cardiovascular events and represent a potential cofounder in some studies.[53]

TRITON-TIMI: Trial to Assess Improvement in Therapeutic Outcomes by Optimizing Platelet Inhibition with Prasugrel

More evidence against the clinical significance of PPI-clopidogrel interaction comes from a post-hoc analysis performed by O'Donoghue et al comparing PPI use versus non-PPI use in the double-blind randomized phase 3 TRITON-TIMI trial.[54] This trial consisted of 13,608 patients with ACS who were randomly assigned to clopidogrel or prasugrel and PPI use. There was no association of an increased risk of the primary endpoint for patients on clopidogrel, irrespective of choice of PPI (HR 0.98, 95% CI 0.84-1.14, p=0.80). Patients with a history of peptic ulcer disease and lower baseline hemoglobin at time of randomization were more likely to receive a PPI. The authors did point out important limitations of their study, which included non-randomization of PPI use and a post-hoc design that may contain the potential for cofounders. Despite these limitations, their analysis serves to support the potential disconnect between findings from platelet studies and the observed clinical significance.[54]

Meta-Analysis

The most recent and comprehensive systematic review on the potential PPI-clopidogrel interaction further highlights the ambiguity between laboratory studies and clinical significance, adding to the difficulty in creating a single consensus based on current data. Focks et al reported that among laboratory studies, 70% (7/10) of healthy participants were found to have a significant reduction in platelet inhibition by clopidogrel and that for clinical studies, 61% (11/18) of patients were found to have a significant reduction.[55] More importantly, however, their analysis of 33 clinical studies showed wide heterogeneity amongst the studies with risk ratios ranging from 0.64-4.58 with the better designed prospective, randomized control trials showing the least supporting evidence. Additionally, confounding the data from the clinical studies was the wide variety of studies types applied: 2 randomized control trials, 7 prospective registries, 19 retrospective cohort studies, 3 post hoc analyses, and 2 case controlled. Taken together, the authors concluded that "considering the firmly and thoroughly established relative benefit of about 20% from the addition of clopidogrel to aspirin, we feel that the reported magnitudes of increased risk cannot be (solely) attributed to the use of PPIs in many of these studies." This same viewpoint is also shared in a current review of the topic from two leading cardiology experts, who conclude "the pharmacokinetic and pharmacodynamic effects of PPIs on the currently available antiplatelets agents do not conclusively result in a clinically significant drug-drug interaction."[56]

VI. Guidance

Alternative Treatment Options

Antacids

Carbonate / Bicarbonate

Most commonly calcium bicarbonate, these antacids work by neutralizing the effects of hydrochloric acid. Side effects of calcium carbonate include hypercalcemia, metabolic alkalosis, and milk-alkali syndrome. There have been no studies to date demonstrating any drug-drug interactions between calcium bicarbonate and clopidogrel.[57]

Aluminum Hydroxide

An inorganic salt which acts by neutralizing hydrochloric acid, aluminum hydroxide is slowly solubilized to react with hydrochloric acid to form water and aluminum chloride. There have been no studies to date demonstrating any drug-drug interactions between aluminum hydroxide and clopidogrel.[58]

H2 Receptor Antagonists

The H-2 receptor antagonists are a class of drugs which block the action of histamine on the parietal cell. Normally when histamine binds to the H2 receptor on the parietal cell, gastric acid (hydrochloric acid) and intrinsic factor are released. In blocking the receptor, the production of acid by parietal cells in the stomach is diminished.[59]

Nizatidine (Axid®)

Axid is an H2 receptor antagonist that does not interfere with the CP450 enzyme system, thus does not interact with concomitant administration with clopidogrel. Some data has shown, however, an increase in serum salicylate levels when patients were given very high doses of aspirin daily (3,900 mg) in addition to nizatidine (150 mg twice daily).[60]

Famotidine (Pepcid®)

At present, studies to date with famotidine have shown no significant interference with the CP450 enzyme system. Thus, current manufacturer recommendations are that famotidine is safe to use simultaneously with other medications.[61]

Cimetidine (Tagamet®)

Cimetidine inhibits multiple enzymes within the CYP450 enzyme system, namely CYP1A2, CYP2C9, CYP2D6, CYP3A3/A4 and CYP2C18.[62] Inhibition of the CP450 enzyme system may potentiate the antiplatelet activity of clopidogrel, especially in those patients with the reduced function CYP2C19 alleles. Special consideration should be taken when co-administering clopidogrel and cimetidine.[63]

Ranitidine (Zantac®)

Ranitidine acts an inhibitor of the CP450 enzyme pathway.[64] A recent study collected serum from 15 patients with stable coronary artery disease. Each patient was administered 600 mg of clopidogrel as a loading dose and their responsiveness was assessed 24 hours later via the $P2Y_{12}$ specific platelet-reactivity-index (PRI) and light transmittance aggregometry in the presence and absence of ranitidine (400ng/ml). The study showed ranitidine significantly enhanced their responsiveness to ADP and impaired inhibition of $P2Y_{12}$, demonstrating a significant interaction between ranitidine and clopidogrel.[65]

Formulary/Cost

Currently, there are an estimated 50 million people prescribed Plavix at an average cost of approximately $200 per month.[66] On May 17th, 2012 the FDA approved generic formulation of Plavix, now available as clopidogrel.[67] With generic out-of-pocket expenses costing approximately $10 per month as a copay with insurance or $40 per month out-of-pocket without insurance, Plavix manufacturers, Bristol-Myers Squibb and Sanofi-Aventis, are offering a Plavix Choice Program, which will cap the costs of out of pocket expenses for branded Plavix at $37 per month.[68] Additionally, generic costs may further decrease as there are plans for six additional generics in the standard 75 mg dose and four additional in the 300 mg dose.

Dose Timing

Another important aspect for determining the clinical significance of the reported clopidogrel-PPI interaction is to determine whether timing of treatment impacts the pharmacokinetic interaction between clopidogrel and PPIs. To address this, a 4-arm study was conducted among 282 healthy subjects to investigate the potential interaction between clopidogrel (300 mg loading dose followed by a 75 mg daily maintenance dose) and high-dose omeprazole at 80 mg daily. The second arm of the study was to determine whether administering clopidogrel and omeprazole 12 hours apart could mitigate the interaction, if any at all. This double-blind randomized study consisted of 72 healthy subjects (demographics shown below with arm-2 highlighted in figure 1) in which they were administered either clopidogrel (300 mg loading dose followed by 75 mg daily maintenance dose) or placebo in addition to omeprazole 80 mg daily 12 hours apart. Vasodilator-simulated phosphoprotein phosphorylation-platelet reactivity index (VASP-PRI) was used to determine the affect on platelet aggregation with higher values corresponding to less platelet inhibition.

As compared to administration of clopidogrel alone, administration of omeprazole 12 hours after being given a loading dose of clopidogrel increased the exposure of unchanged clopidogrel by 19% ($p=0.012$) and decreased the exposure of its active metabolite (clop-H4) by 53% ($p<0.001$). On day 5 (having been administered loading dose of clopidogrel and 4 days of maintenance dose clopidogrel with each dose being followed 12 hours later

	Study 1[a] (N=72)	Study 2[b] (N=72)	Study 3[c] (N=72)	Study 4[d] (N=66)
Age, mean (SD) years	33.8 (10.0)	32.0 (8.8)	34.7 (14.5)	32.3 (8.9)
Men, n(%)	60 (83.3)	69 (95.8)	48 (66.7)	66 (100)
Race, n(%)				
Caucasian/White	44 (66.1)	71 (98.6)	51 (70.8)	52 (78.8)
Black	8 (11.1)	1 (3.9)	6 (8.3)	11 (16.7)
Asian	1(1.4)	0 (0.0)	3 (4.2)	2 (3.0)
Other	19 (26.4)	0 (0.0)	12 (16.7)	1 (1.5)
Weight, mean (SD) kg	75.9 (10.8)	72.6 (9.3)	70.3 (10.8)	78.28 (9.5)
Height, mean (SD) cm	171.7 (9.3)	167.5 (6.8)	171.9 (9.4)	175.5 (6.5)
Body mass index, mean (SD) kg/m^2	25.7 (2.8)	25.9 (2.4)	23.8 (2.9)	25.4 (2.6)

[a]Clopidogrel (300mg loading dose), 75mg maintenance dose and omeprazole 80mg/day administered simultaneously
[b]Clopidogrel (300mg loading dose), 75mg maintenance dose and omeprazole 80mg/day administered 12 hours apart
[c]Clopidogrel (600mg loading dose), 150mg maintenance dose and omeprazole 80mg/day administered simultaneously
[d]Clopidogrel (300mg loading dose), 75mg maintenance dose and pantoprazole 80mg/day administered simultaneously

Figure 4. Four-arm study conducted to determine whether timing of treatment impacts the pharmacokinetic interaction between clopidogrel and PPIs.

with omeprazole) the exposure of unchanged clopidogrel increased by 37% ($p<0.001$) whereas clop-H4 exposure decreased by 47% ($p<0.001$). The chart below depicts the interaction between clopidogrel and omeprazole as measured by VASP-PRI on days 1, 2 and 5. This study proved that the interactions between clopidogrel and omeprazole were unaffected by dose sequence.[69]

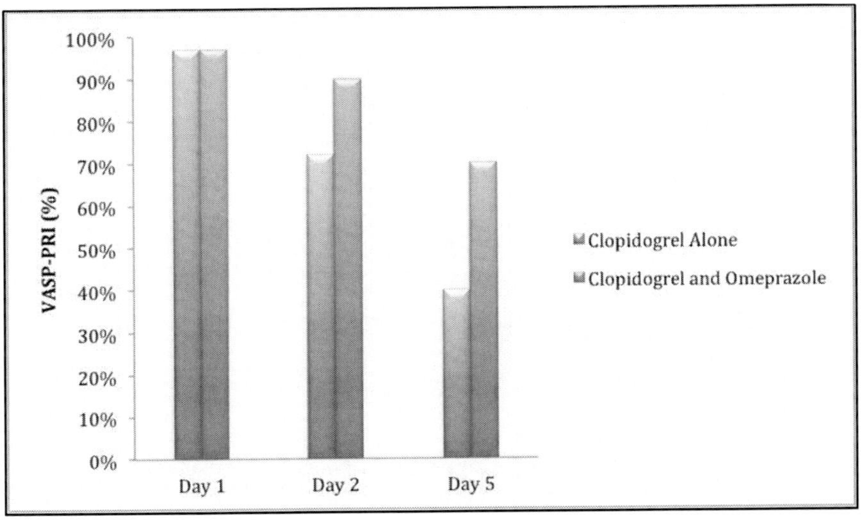

Figure 5. Depicts the interaction between clopidogrel and omeprazole as measured by VASP-PRI on days 1, 2 and 5.

Additionally, a prospective, randomized, crossover study was conducted in 20 healthy volunteers to assess the impact of high dose pantoprazole therapy on clopidogrel metabolism and whether administered concomitantly or staggered would alter the pharmacodynamics effects. Subjects were assigned to receive pantoprazole (80 mg daily) concomitantly or staggered by 8 to 12 hours for one week with clopidogrel (600 mg loading dose followed by a 75 mg daily maintenance dose). The results (shown below) indicate that high doses of pantoprazole, irrespective of timing of drug administration, do not alter the pharmacodynamics effects of clopidogrel.[70]

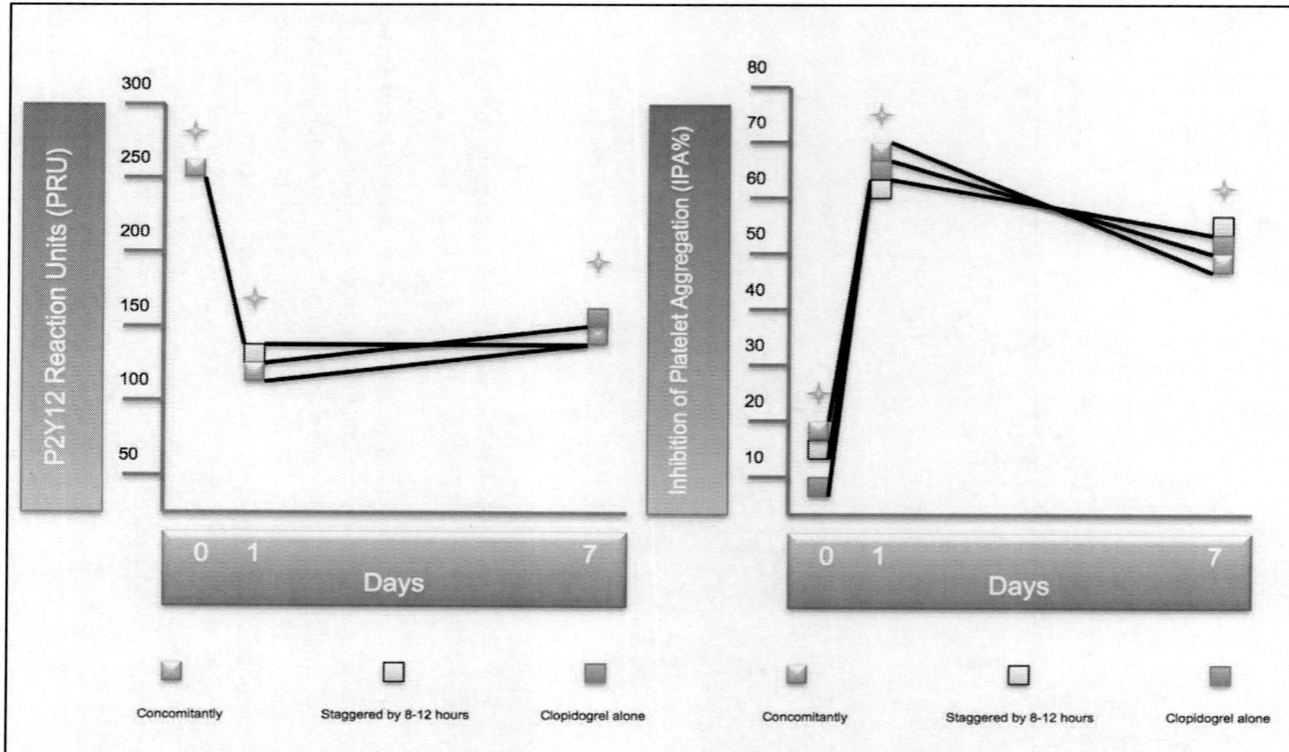

Figure 6. Results of study to assess the impact of high dose pantoprazole therapy on clopidogrel metabolism and whether administered concomitantly or staggered would alter the pharmacodynamics effects.

CONCLUSION

Clopidogrel is a mainstay in cardiac patients suffering from ACS and in those with a recent MI as a preventative for future cardiovascular events. A known risk of clopidogrel is the possibility of a GI bleed and consequently many patients prescribed an antisecretory agent. Proton pump inhibitors have been shown to be the most efficacious in its antisecretory effect in these patients, however, several studies have shown a significant pharmacodynamic interaction between PPIs and clopidogrel.

Focused around the CYP2C19 isoenzyme, several factors are thought to play a role in the metabolism from clopidogrel to its active metabolite. While all PPIs have been shown to affect the CYP2C19 enzyme to some degree, the FDA has recommended avoiding concomitant use of clopidogrel with omeprazole or esomeprazole. Current guidelines state that pantoprazole, lansoprazole or dexlansoprazole are less likely to affect metabolism of clopidogrel to be active metabolite and are safe to co-administer. The newer data on a possible interaction with pantoprazole, however, warrant further evaluation[40].

Despite FDA recommendations, numerous studies have highlighted the difficulty in applying data from platelet aggregation studies into the clinical setting. Additionally, the most recent meta-analysis suggests that no definitive statement on the impact of PPIs on clopidogrel activity can be concluded at this time, rather physicians should weigh patients on a case-by case-basis and keep PPIs where clinically justified.

SUMMARY POINTS

1. Clopidogrel is a pro-drug that is metabolized to its active metabolite via the CYP450 enzyme pathway, namely the CYP2C19 enzyme.
2. Genetic polymorphisms (in particular CYP2C19*2 reduced function allele) and medications (i.e. PPIs) affect the CYP2C19 enzyme which result in reduced platelet inhibition.
3. Omeprazole and esomeprazole have been shown as having the most significant impact on the CYP450 enzyme pathway in platelet aggregation studies and are not recommended to be in used in conjunction with clopidogrel. The FDA has taken steps to ensure that

the PPIs co-prescribed with clopidogrel are limited to pantoprazole, lansoprazole and dexlansoprazole.

4. In contrast to the FDA recommendations, numerous high-profile clinical trials (i.e. COGENT, CREDO) have documented no clinically significant interaction between PPIs and clopidogrel.
5. A study determining whether administering clopidogrel and omeprazole 12 hours apart could mitigate the interaction proved that the interactions between clopidogrel and omeprazole was unaffected by dose sequence.
6. H2 receptor antagonists offer an alternative to proton pump inhibitors albeit less efficacious, however, cimetidine and ranitidine may also cause significant interaction with CYP2C19 and should not be used in conjunction with clopidogrel therapy.
7. In the future, the role of pharmacogenomic testing or platelet function testing in managing therapy with clopidogrel and PPIs will need to be established.

REFERENCES

[1] Go, AS; Mozaffarian, D; Roger, VL; et al. Heart disease and stroke statistics - 2013 update a report from the American Heart Association. *Circulation*, 2013; 127.

[2] Levine, GN; Bates, ER; Blakenship, JC; et al. 2011 ACCF/AHA/SCAI guideline for percutaneous coronary intervention: a report of the American College of Cardiology Foundation/American Heart Association task force on practice guidelines and the Society for Cardiovascular Angiographs and Interventions. *J Am Coll Cardiol.*, 2011, 58(24), e44-122.

[3] Goodwin, MM; Desilets, AR; Willet, KC. Thienopyridines in acute coronary syndrome. *Ann Pharmacother.*, 2011, 45(2), 207-217.

[4] PLAVIX® (clopidogrel bisulfate) Prescribing Information." *Sanofi-Aventis Prescription Products*. Sanofi-Aventis; n.d. Web. 18 Dec. 2012. <products.sanofi.us/plavix/plavix.html>.

[5] Abraham, NS; Graham, DY. NSAIDs and gastrointestinal complications: new clinical challenges. *Expert Opin Pharmacother.*, 2005, 6, 2681-9.

[6] Abraham, NS; Hlatky, MA; Antman, EM; et al. ACCF/ACG/AHA 2010 Expert consensus document on the concomitant use of proton pump

inhibitors and thienopyridines: a focused update of the ACCF/ACG/ AHA 2008 expert consensus document on reducing the gastrointestinal risks of antiplatelet therapy and NSAID use. *Am J Gastroenterol.*, 2010, 105(12), 2233-59.

[7] http://www.fda.gov/Drugs/DrugSafety/PostmarketDrugSafetyInformationforPatientsandProviders/DrugSafetyInformationforHeathcareProfessionals/ucm079520.htm

[8] http://www.fda.gov/Drugs/DrugSafety/PostmarketDrugSafetyInformationforPatientsandProviders/DrugSafetyInformationforHeathcareProfessionals/ucm190784.htm

[9] Maloney, JP; Silliman, CC; Ambruso, DR; et al. In vitro release of vascular endothelial growth factor during platelet aggregation. *Am J Physiol.*, 1998, 275(3 Pt 2), H1054-1061.

[10] Ma, L; Elliott, SN; Cirino, G; et al. Platelets modulate gastric ulcer healing: role of endostatin and vascular endothelial growth factor release. *PNAS.*, 2001, 98(11), 6470-6475.

[11] Van, HA; Depre, M; Wynants, K; et al. Effect of clopidogrel on naproxen-induced gastrointestinal blood loss in healthy volunteers. *Drug Metabol Drug Interact.*, 1998,14,193-205.

[12] Yusuf, F; Zhao, F; Mehta, SR; et al. Effects of clopidogrel in addition to aspirin in patients with acute coronary syndromes without ST-segment elevation. *N Engl J Med.*, 2001, 345(7), 494-502

[13] Connolly, SJ; Pogue, J; Hart, RG; et al. Effect of clopidogrel added to aspirin in patients with atrial fibrillation. *N Engl J Med.*, 2009, 360(20), 2066-78.

[14] Moukarbel, GK; Signorovitch, JE; Pfeffer, MA; et al. Gastrointestinal bleeding in high risk survivors of myocardial infarction: the VALIANT trial. *Eur Heart J.*, 2009, 30(18), 2226-32.

[15] Garcia Rodruigez, LA; Lin, KJ; Hernandez-Diaz, S; Johansson, S. Risk of upper gastrointestinal bleeding with low-dose acetylsalicylic acid alone and in combination with clopidogrel and other medications. *Circulation*, 2011, 123, 1108-1115

[16] Arroyo, RC; Polo-Thomas, M; Roncales, MP; et al. Lower GI bleeding is more common than upper among patients on dual anti-platelet therapy: long-term follow-up of a cohort of patients commonly using PPI co-therapy. Heart, 2012, 98, 718-723.

[17] Abraham, NS; Hlatky, MA; Antman, EM; et al. ACCF/ACG/AHA 2010 Expert consensus document on the concomitant use of proton pump inhibitors and thienopyridines: a focused update of the ACCF/ACG/

AHA 2008 expert consensus document on reducing the gastrointestingal risks of antiplatelet therapy and NSAID use. *Am J Gastroenterol.*, 2010, 105(12), 2233-59.

[18] Grines, CL; Bonow, RO; Casey, DE; Jr.; et al. Prevention of premature discontinuation of dual antiplatelet therapy in patients with coronary artery stents: a science advisory from the American Heart Association; American College of Cardiology; Society for Cardiovascular Angiography and Interventions; American College of Surgeons; and American Dental Association; with representation from the American College of Physicians. *Circulation.*, 2007, 115(6), 813-8.

[19] Iakovou, I; Schmidt, T; Bonizzoni, E; et al. Incidence; predictors; and outcome of thrombosis after successful implantation of drug-eluting stents. JAMA, 2005, 293, 2126–30.

[20] Whellan, DL; Goldstein, JL; Scheiman, JM; et al. Treatment continuation and cardiovascular safety of antiplatelet therapy with PA32540; a tablet with enteric-coated aspirin and immediate-release omeprazole: results of two 6-month; phase 3 studies. Poster presented at the American Heart Association Scientific Sessions, 2012, November 3-7; Los Angeles; CA.

[21] Sangkuhl, K; Klein, KE; Altman, RB. Clopidogrel pathway. *Pharmacogenet Genomics.*, 2010, 20(7), 463-65.

[22] Savi, P; Combalbert, J; Gaich C; et al. The antiaggregating activity of clopidogrel is due to a metabolic activation by the hepatic cytochrome P450-1A. *Thromb Haemost.*, 1994, 72, 313-7.

[23] Kazui, M; Nishiya, Y; Ishizuka, T; Hagihara, K; Farid, NA; Okazaki, O; et al. Identification of the human cytochrome P450 enzymes involved in the two oxidative steps in the bioactivation of clopidogrel to its pharmacologically active metabolite. *Drug Metab Dispos.*, 2010, 38, 92–99.

[24] Schomig, As. Ticagrelor - is there a need for a new player in the antiplatelet-therapy field? *N Engl J Med.*, 2009, 361(11), 1108-11.

[25] Tauber, D; von Beckerath, N; Grimberg, G; et al. Impact of p-glycoprotein on clopidogrel absorption. *Clin Pharmacol Ther.*, 2006, 80, 486-501.

[26] Pauli-Magnus, C; Rekersbrink, S; Klotz, U; Fromm, MF. Interaction of omeprazole; lansoprazole and pantoprazole with P-glycoprotein. *Naunyn Schmiedebergs Arch Pharmacol*, 2001, 364, 551-7.

[27] Horstrup, K; Jablonka, B; Hönig-Liedl, M; et al. Phosphorylation of focal adhesion vasodilator-stimulated phosphoprotein at Ser157 in intact

human platelets correlates with fibrinogen receptor inhibition. *Eur J Biochem.*, 1994, 225, 21-27.

[28] Norgard, NB; Mathwes, KD; Wall, GC. Drug-drug interaction between clopidogrel and the proton pump inhibitors. *Ann Pharmacother.*, 2009, 43(7), 1266-74.

[29] Savi, P; Pereillo, JM; Uzabiaga, MF; et al. Identification and biological ac-tivity of the active metabolite of clopidogrel. *Thromb Haemost*, 2000, 84, 891-6.

[30] Desta, Z; Zhao, X; Shin, JG; Flockhart DA. Clinical significance of the cytochrome P450 2C19 genetic polymorphism. *Clin Pharmacokinet*, 2002, 41, 913-58.

[31] Mega, JL; Close, SL; Wiviott, SD; et al. Cytochrome P450 polymorphisms and response to clopidogrel. *N Engl Med J.*, 2009, 360, 354-62.

[32] Mega, JL; Close, SL; Wiviott, SD; et al. Cytochrome P450 genetic polymorphisms and the response to prasugrel: relationship to pharmacokinetic; pharmacodynamic; and clinical outcomes. *Circulation.*, 2009, 119, 2553-2560.

[33] Harmsze, AM; Van werkum, JW; Souverein, PC; et al. Combined influence of proton-pump inhibitors; calcium channel blockers and CYP2C19*2 on on-treatment platelet reactivity and on the occurrence of atherothrombotic events after percutaneous coronary intervention. *J Thromb Haemost.*, 2011, 9, 1892-1901.

[34] Mega, JL; Close, SL; Wiviott, SD; et al. Genetic variants in ABCB1; CYP2C19; and cardiovascular outcomes following treatment with clopidogrel and prasugrel. *Lancet.*, 2010, 376(9749), 1312-1319.

[35] AztraZeneca, Prilosec. "*PRILOSEC® (omeprazole) Delayed-Release Capsules Prescribing Information.* AztraZeneca; n.d. Web. 18 Dec. 2012. <www1.astrazeneca-us.com/pi/Prilosec.pdf>.

[36] NEXIUM® (esomeprazole magnesium) Presribing Informatiom ."*Heartburn Relief | NEXIUM® (esomeprazole magnesium) - The Purple Pill.* AztraZeneca; n.d. Web. 18 Dec. 2012. <http://www. purplepill.com/>.

[37] PREVACID® (lansoprazole) Prescribing Information." *Takeda Pharmaceuticals U.S.A.; Inc.* Takeda Pharmaceuticals; n.d. Web. 18 Dec. 2012. <http://www.takeda.us/products/default.aspx>.

[38] DEXILANT® (dexlansoprazole) Prescribing Information." *Takeda Pharmaceuticals U.S.A.; Inc.*. N.p.; n.d. Web. 18 Dec. 2012. <http://www. takeda.us/products/default.aspx>.

[39] PROTONIX® (pantoprazole) Prescribing Information." *Pharmaceutical Company | Pfize: the world's largest research-based pharmaceutical company*. Pfizer; n.d. Web. 18 Dec. 2012. <http://www. pfizer. com/ products/#A>.

[40] Parri, MS; Gianetti, J; Dushpanova, A; et al. Pantoprazole significantly interferes with antiplatelet effect of clopidogrel: results of a pilot randomized control trial. *Int J Cardiol*., 2012. Epub ahead of print.

[41] Gilard, M; Arnaud, B; Cornily, J-C; et al. Influence of omeprazole on the antiplatelet action of clopidogrel associated with aspirin: the randomized; double-blind OCLA (Omeprazole Clopidogrel Aspirin) study. *J Am Coll Cardiol*., 2008, 51, 256-260.

[42] O'Donoghue, ML; Braunwald, E; Antman, EM; et al. Pharmacodynamic effect and clinical efficacy of clopidogrel and prasugrel with or without a proton-pump inhibitor: an analysis of two randomised trials. *Lancet*., 2009, 374(9694), 989-97.

[43] Frelinger, AL; Lee, RD; Mulford, DJ; et al. A randomized; 2-period; crossover design study to assess the effects of dexlansoprazole; lansoprazole; esomeprazole; and omeprazole on the steady-state pharmacokinetics and pharmacodynamics of clopidogrel in healthy volunteers. *J Am Coll Cardiol*., 2012, 59(14), 1304-11.

[44] Déry, JP. editor. SPICE: A prospective; randomized trial of four antacid strategies in patients receiving clopidogrel. Transcatheter Cardiovascular Therapeutics 2011 November 9; San Francisco; CA.

[45] Siller-Matula, JM; Spiel, AO; Lang, IM; et al. Effects of pantoprazole and esomeprazole on platelet inhibition by clopidogrel. *Am Heart J*., 2009,157, 148.e1-148.e5.

[46] Tunggal, P; Ng, F; Lam, K; et al. Effect of esomeprazole versus famotidine on platelet inhibition by clopidogrel: a double-blind; randomized trial. *Am Heart J*., 2011, 162(5), 870-4.

[47] Humphries, TJ. Famotidine: a notable lack of drug interactions. *Scand J Gastroenterol Suppl*., 1987, 143, 55-60.

[48] Andersson, T; Nagy, P; Niazi, M; et al. Impact of omeprazole (OME); esomeprazole (ESO) +/- acetylsalicylic acid (ASA) and lansoprazole (LAN) on the pharmacodynamics (PD) and pharmacokinetics (PK) of clopidogrel in healthy volunteers. *European heart journal*., 2012, 33 (Abstract supplement), 343.

[49] Bhatt, DL; Cryer, BL; Contant, CF; et al. Clopidogrel with or without omeprazole in coronary artery disease. *N Engl J Med*., 2010, 363, 1909-17.

[50] Kleinrock, M. The use of medicines in the United States: review of 2010. IMS Institute for Healthcare Informatics. April 2011.

[51] Li, XQ; Anderson, TB; Ahlstrom, M; Weidolf, L. Comparison of inhibitory effects of the proton-inhibiting drugs omeprazole; esomeprazole; lansoprazole; pantoprazole; and rabeprazole on human cytochrome P450 activities. *Drug Metab Dispos.*, 2004, 32(8), 821-7.

[52] Dunn, SP; Macaulay, TE; Brennan, DM; et al. Abstract 3999: Baseline proton pump inhibitor use is associated with increased cardiovascular events with and without the use of clopidogrel in the CREDO trial. *Circulation.*, 2008, 118, S815.

[53] Goodman, et al. Association of proton pump inhibitor use on cardiovascular outcome with clopidogrel and ticagrelor: insights from PLATO. *Circulation*, 2012, 125(8), 978-86.

[54] O'Donoghue, ML; Braunwald, E; Antman, EM; et al. Pharmacodynamic effect and clinical efficacy of clopidogrel and prasugrel with or without a proton-pump inhibitor: an analysis of two randomised trials. *Lancet.*, 2009, 374(9694), 989-97.

[55] Focks, JJ; Brouwer, MA; van Oijen, MGH; et al. Concomitant use of clopidogrel and proton pump inhibitors: impact on platelet function and clinical outcome – a systematic review. *Heart.*, 2012. Doi: 10.1136/heartjnl-2012-302371.

[56] Depta, JP; Bhatt, DL. Antiplatelet therapy and proton pump inhibition: cause for concern? *Curr Opin Cariol.*, 2012, 27, 642-650.

[57] Calcium Carbonate (OTC) Pharmacology. "*Medscape: Medscape Access*. N.p.; n.d. Web. 31 Dec. 2012. <http://reference.medscape.com/drug/caltrate-600-os-cal-500-d-calcium-carbonate-341983#10>.

[58] Aluminum Hydroxide (OTC) Pharmacology ."*Medscape: Medscape Access*. N.p.; n.d. Web. 31 Dec. 2012. <http://reference.medscape.com/drug/mylanta-mygel-aluminum-hydroxide-magnesium-hydroxide-simethicone-341982#10>.

[59] Bowen; R.. "Histamine and Histamine Receptors." *arbl.cvmbs.colostate.edu*. N.p.; n.d. Web. 31 Dec. 2012. <http://www.vivo.colostate.edu/hbooks/pathphys/endocrine/otherendo/histamine.html>.

[60] Axid Official FDA information; side effects and uses.." *Drugs.com | Prescription Drug Information; Interactions & Side Effects*. N.p.; n.d. Web. 31 Dec. 2012. <http://www.drugs.com/pro/axid.html>.

[61] PEPCID ® (Famotidine) Prescribing Information." *Merck. A global healthcare leader working to help the world be well.*. Merck & Co.;

INC. (USA); n.d. Web. 2 Jan. 2013. <http://www.merck.com/product/usa/pi_circulars/p/products_p.html>

[62] "TAGAMET® PRODUCT INFORMATION (cimetidine). "*GlaxoSmithKline*. GlaxoSmithKline; n.d. Web. 2 Jan. 2013. <www.gsk.com.au/resources.ashx/prescriptionmedicinesproductschilddataproinfo/843/FileName/1BF361428971B19DA2CEF2E3EAD3BE09/PI_Tagamet.pdf>.

[63] Shuldiner, Alan R; et al. Association of cytochrome P450 2C19 genotype with the antiplatelet effect and clinical efficacy of clopidogrel therapy. JAMA. 2009; 302 (8), 849-857.

[64] ZANTAC ® (ranitidine hydrochloride) Prescribing Information." *GlaxoSmithKline*. GlaxoSmithKline; n.d. Web. 2 Jan. 2013. <us.gsk.com/products/assets/us_zantac.pdf>.

[65] Schäfer, A; et al. "The H(2)-receptor antagonist ranitidine interferes with clopidogrel-mediated P2Y(12) inhibition in platelets. Pharmacol Res., 2010, 62(4), 352-6.

[66] Strawbridge, Holly. "Wallets rejoice as Plavix goes generic - Harvard Health Publications." *Harvard Health Publications*. N.p.; n.d. Web. 31 Dec. 2012. <http://www.health.harvard.edu/blog/wallets-rejoice-as-plavix-goes-generic-201205214727>.

[67] http://www.fda.gov/NewsEvents/Newsroom/PressAnnouncements/ucm304489.htm

[68] Corbett Dooren; Jennifer. "FDA Approves Generic Versions of Plavix - WSJ.com."*The Wall Street Journal*. N.p.; n.d. Web. 31 Dec. 2012. <http://online.wsj.com/article/SB10001424052702303448404577410464001441678.html>.

[69] Angiolillo, D; et al. Differential Effects of Omeprazole and Pantoprazole on the Pharmacodynamics and Pharmacokinetics of Clopidogrel in Healthy Subjects: Randomized; Placebo-Controlled; Crossover Comparison Studies. *Clin Pharmacol Ther.*, 2011, 89, 65-74.

[70] Luis Ferreiro, MD; José; et al. Pharmacodynamic Evaluation of Pantoprazole Therapy on Clopidogrel Effects Clinical Perspective. *Circulation*., 2011, 4, 273-279.

In: Clopidogrel
Editors: J. P. Alesci and A. Victorino
ISBN: 978-1-62948-336-8
© 2014 Nova Science Publishers, Inc.

Chapter 7

Perioperative Management of Clopidogrel in Urological Surgery

N. F. Davis*[*], *J. C. Forde and H. D. Flood
Department of Urology, University of Limerick Teaching Hospital,
Co Limerick, Ireland

Abstract

Introduction: There has been a significant increase in the volume of urological patients on daily clopidogrel therapy that require invasive elective urological procedures. In the present chapter we sought to assess current scientific evidence for appropriately managing this patient cohort during the perioperative period.

Methods: A literature search for English language publications using the PubMed® and Embase® databases was performed. Keywords included "clopidogrel," "perioperative management" and "urological surgery." A total of 148 articles were analysed, of which 86 were suitable for analysis based on clinical relevance and importance of content.

Results: Clopidogrel is compulsory for 4-6 weeks after insertion of bare metal stents (BMS). It is also mandatory for up to 12 months after insertion of drug-eluting stents (DES). Elective urological surgery must be either delayed beyond these waiting periods or performed with patients

[*] Corresponding author: Niall F. Davis, Department of Urology, University of Limerick Teaching Hospital, Dooradoyle, Co Limerick, Ireland, Email: nialldavis2001@yahoo.com.

receiving daily clopidogrel as withdrawal of the agent results in a five- to ten-fold increase in the risk of postoperative MI, stent thrombosis or death. The risk of perioperative surgical bleeding is increased by 50% in patients where clopidogrel is continued.

Conclusion: The risk of cardiovascular morbidity (i.e. coronary thrombosis) when clopidogrel is discontinued before elective urological surgery is generally higher than the risk of perioperative bleeding when the agent is continued. It is imperative that urologists are familiar with standardised guidelines if this increasing patient cohort is to receive optimal perioperative management.

1. Introduction

Clopidogrel is a frequently prescribed antithrombotic agent that has been shown to be effective in treating a number of common cardiovascular conditions ('Collaborative meta-analysis of randomised' 2002). Despite its widespread prevalence, evidence-based recommendations on perioperative management protocols for urological procedures are lacking (Giannarini et al. 2007). Patient-specific risk factors are taken into account on an individual basis and a clinical decision is invariably made based on these risk factors by the operating urological surgeon. This may result in a broad spectrum of procedure-specific management policies that range from continuing clopidogrel during the perioperative period to discontinuing and recommencing the agent a number of weeks pre- and postoperatively. Significant perioperative risks are associated with both perioperative policies. Continuation predisposes to intraoperative and postoperative bleeding (Burger et al. 2005) while cessation predisposes to an increased risk of stroke, myocardial infarction (MI) and cardiac death (Heit 2001, Connor and Wingate 1999). The objective of this chapter is to investigate appropriate management strategies for clopidogrel in urological surgery during the perioperative period.

2. Mechanism of Action

Platelets are anucleate cells produced from megakaryocytes in the bone marrow and their primary function is to stop bleeding after tissue trauma and vascular injury. The physiological response at the site of vascular injury involves platelet activation, adhesion and release of various autocrine and paracrine mediators like thromboxane A2, epinephrine and adenosine diphosphate (ADP) (Kapoor 2008). These mediators stimulate a host-derived platelet response which results in aggregation and formation of haemostatic plugs (Davi and Patrono 2007). Platelets also play a role in the development of atherosclerotic plaques and antiplatelet agents are frequently prescribed by clinicians to inhibit this pathological process.

Clopidogrel is a thienopyridine that is oxidized by hepatic cytochromes into an active metabolite that has a plasma elimination half-life of 8 hours. The agent acts by covalently binding to a cysteine residue of the ADP/P2Y12 platelet receptor (O'Riordan et al. 2009) and blockage of this receptor irreversibly inhibits platelet aggregation is a dose dependent manner.

Therefore, platelets are affected for the remainder of their life span which is usually 7-10 days (Kaushansky 1998, Eberli et al. 2010). Usually, 80% of platelets have recovered normal aggregation after 7 days of cessation. Another option is to start with a loading dose of 300–600 mg and then shift to 75 mg/day. In this way, platelet inhibition effect is demonstrable within a few hours (Eberli et al. 2010). Ticlopidine, another drug that belongs to the same family as clopidogrel, has now been virtually abandoned because of the frequency of side effects, which include neutropenia (1-2.4%) and thrombotic thrombocytopenic purpura (1 in 3000)(Bertrand et al. 2000, Muller et al. 2001).

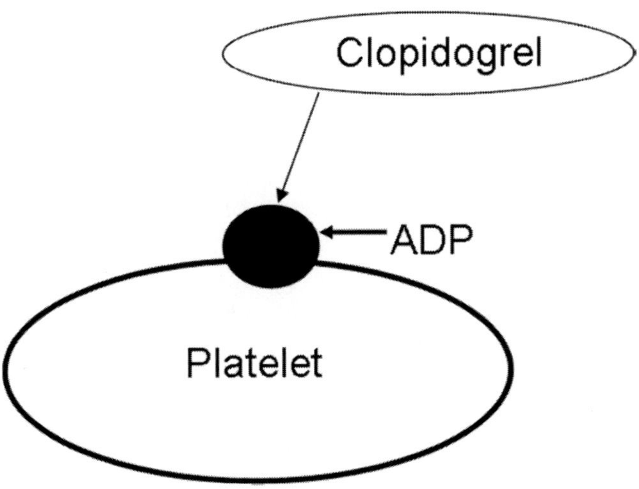

Figure 1. Mechanism of action of clopidogrel.

3. Indications for Clopidogrel

Clopidogrel has a defined role in relation to percutaneous coronary intervention (PCI) (Steinhubl et al. 2002, Ringleb et al. 2004, Bhatt et al. 2001, Bhatt et al. 2006, Bhatt et al. 2002, Mehta et al. 2001, Kastrati et al. 2004) with the CURE study demonstrating the benefit of adding clopidogrel to aspirin (additional 10% relative risk reduction) rather than using aspirin alone in patients with non-ST-segment elevation acute coronary intervention (ACS) or unstable angina (Yusuf et al. 2001, Eagle et al. 2002).

It is now well established that the duration of dual antiplatelet (i.e. aspirin and clopidogrel) treatment among patients with PCIs and coronary stents is 4–6 weeks after bare metal stents (BMS) implantation, 3 months after sirolimus drug-eluting stents (DES) (CypherTM) implantation, 6 months after paclitaxel DES (TaxusTM AchieveTM, V-flexTM, CoStarTM) implantation, and 3–6 months for second generation DES (zotarolimus; EndeavorTM; everolimus; Xience VTM) implantation (Smith et al. 2006b, Albaladejo et al. 2006, Silber et al. 2005, Smith et al. 2006a, Serruys et al. 2006). Notably, the current Food and Drug Administration (FDA) recommendation is to continue taking both aspirin and clopidogrel for a minimum 12 months after DES (Serruys et al. 2006). A recent advisory from the American Heart Association, American College of Cardiology, and the American College of Surgeons also emphasises the importance of 12 months of dual antiplatelet therapy after insertion of a DES because of the risk of late stent stenosis due to delayed endothelialisation (Grines et al. 2007). Furthermore, patients who are resistant to aspirin (up to 10%) have higher rates of cardiovascular events and can also benefit from clopidogrel therapy (O'Riordan et al. 2009).

Surgeons are more likely to encounter DES as several notable clinical trials have demonstrated that DES are associated with significant reductions in the risks of restenosis and need for revascularization, as compared with use of BMS (Stettler et al. 2007). Therefore, DES are more widely used for PCI in clinical practice (Williams et al. 2006). Importantly, there are longer-term studies that suggest that DES are associated with increased rates of late stent thrombosis, death, or myocardial infarction as compared to BMS.(Bavry and Bhatt 2008, Lagerqvist et al. 2007, Nakazawa et al. 2008). It has been proposed that the occurrence of late clinical events may be due to delayed arterial healing after the implantation of DES (Nakazawa et al. 2008).

Table 1. Recommended duration of dual antiplatelet therapy after percutaneous coronary intervention (Eberli et al. 2010)

Indication	Minimum duration
Angioplasty without stenting	2-4 weeks
Bare metal stent (BMS)	4-6 weeks
Myocardial infarction (MI)	3-6 months
Sirolimus drug-eluting stent (DES) dual treatment	3 months
Paclitaxel DES dual treatment	6 months
Second generation DES dual treatment	3-6 months
Unstable acute coronary syndrome (ACS)	12 months
Percutaneous coronary intervention (PCI) with DES	>12 months

4. Premature Withdrawal of Clopidogrel

In general, about 5% of patients within the first year after intracoronary stent placement will undergo non-cardiac surgery (Nuttall et al. 2008). Discontinuation prior to completing 1 year of therapy is considered premature withdrawal and is associated with death rates of 25%-50% (Collet et al. 2006). In patients who have received a DES, a number of studies have described premature interruption of oral antiplatelet therapy as one of the highest risk factors for delayed stent thrombosis (Ong et al. 2005a, Park et al. 2006, Urban et al. 2006, Kuchulakanti et al. 2006, Jeremias et al. 2004, McFadden et al. 2004, Iakovou et al. 2005, Ferrari et al. 2005). In addition, early withdrawal of clopidogrel may promote a rebound prothrombotic effect (Ferrari et al. 2005, Angiolillo et al. 2006). In perioperative patients, this added risk as well as the underlying risk of thromboembolism associated with surgery could be responsible for the high rates of thrombosis seen in patients who stop taking clopidogrel before major urological procedures, particularly after PCI. Recent American guidelines identify the risk of stent thrombosis from premature antiplatelet drug discontinuation in patients with DES is as high 29%. Stent thrombosis causes a sudden withdrawal of bloodflow in a high-output vessel that provides oxygen to a muscle and this leads to high mortality rates (19–45%) (Iakovou et al. 2005, Kaiser et al. 2005, Ong et al. 2005b, Pfisterer et al. 2006, Ferrari et al. 2005). In fact, early withdrawal of clopidogrel is the most significant independent predictor of stent thrombosis (early DES thrombosis) as demonstrated in one study with 2,229 patients with DES and a thrombosis rate of 1.5% during the first year (hazard ratio: 57.13 ($P<0.001$) and mortality rate due to stent thrombosis: 45% (Iakovou et al. 2005). In the BASKET trial, 746 patients (randomly assigned to BMS or DES and surviving 6 months without major events) were followed for a further year after withdrawing clopidogrel at 6 months (Pfisterer et al. 2006). The 18-months rate of re-stenosis was lower in DES compared to BMS (4.5 vs. 8.7%, OR 0.51). However, MI and death rates 7–18 months after stopping clopidogrel were higher with DES than with BMS (4.9 vs. 1.3%, adjusted HR 2.2, P<0.03).

5. Propensity for Bleeding

There are no specific guidelines regarding treatment of bleeding in patients taking clopidogrel; however the agent has a greater propensity to cause bleeding when compared to aspirin. This was initially demonstrated in the CAPRIE study where the incidence of spontaneous intracranial haemorrhage (0.35%, p> 0.05), gastrointestinal bleeding (0.68% $p < 0.05$) and gastrointestinal ulcers (0.68%, p< 0.05) was greater in patients on chronic clopidogrel therapy when compared to aspirin alone ('Collaborative meta-analysis of randomised trials of antiplatelet therapy for prevention of death, myocardial infarction, and stroke in high risk patients' 2002). Notably, the definition of bleeding differs greatly between randomised trials that evaluated clopidogrel and other antiplatelet therapies ('An international randomized trial comparing four thrombolytic strategies for acute myocardial infarction. The GUSTO investigators' 1993, Schulman and Kearon 2005, Chesebro et al. 1987). Eikelboom and Hirsh demonstrated that the absolute increase in risk for major bleeding in randomised trials for clopidogrel was approximately 1% when compared with a placebo (Eikelboom 2006). Their definition for bleeding was based on the International Society on Thrombosis and Haemostasis (Schulman and Kearon 2005). Furthermore, adding clopidogrel to aspirin increased the relative risk of bleeding by up to 50% and bleeding secondary to antiplatelet therapy was independently predictive of adverse clinical outcomes, including myocardial infarction, stroke, and death (Rao et al. 2005, Moscucci et al. 2003).

The antiplatelet effect of clopidogrel may be reversed with platelet transfusions (Vilahur et al. 2007). Platelet transfusion is the only therapeutic option in patients on clopidogrel therapy with severe perioperative haemorrhage. However, there are no clinical studies that clearly demonstrate the advantages of platelet transfusion when limiting a severe perioperative bleed in patients on clopidogrel (Biondi-Zoccai et al. 2006). An important issue to take into consideration prior to an emergency platelet transfusion is the time of the last clopidogrel dose. As clopidogrel has a half-life of 4 hours, its plasma level reaches close to zero after about 12 h (three half-lives) and it is only after 6-8 hours after the last dose of clopidogrel that the transfused platelets will not be significantly affected by the drug (Chassot et al. 2007).

Administration of other antithrombotic agents such as antifibrinolytics (e.g. aprotinin (Levi et al. 1999, Lindvall et al. 2005, Levy 1960, van der Linden et al. 2005, Akowuah et al. 2005), desmopressin acetate (von Heymann et al. 2005, Arom and Emery 1994) and recombinant factor VIIa) are other possible options (Altman et al. 2006). It is unclear whether these agents should be given prophylactically during urgent surgery or only be administered when bleeding arises. In one randomised trial of patients undergoing urgent coronary artery bypass graft, Akowuah *et al.* found that continuing aspirin and clopidogrel therapy with intraoperative aprotinin administration was associated with reduced postoperative blood loss and transfusion requirements compared with stopping the antiplatelet treatment 5 days preoperatively and omitting intraoperative aprotinin (Akowuah et al. 2005).

6. Perioperative Management of Clopidogrel

The most important decision regarding the perioperative management of patients with intracoronary stents is to carefully assess the risks of bleeding associated with continuation of clopidogrel therapy compared with the risks of stent thrombosis when discontinued. Unfortunately, in acute surgical situations it is impossible to differentiate between the presence of BMS or DES unless the patient's medical records are readily available. Perhaps the presence of an 'alert bracelet' on the patient's wrist or a 'stent-specific' identification card would be useful for accurately defining the type of coronary stent in emergency situations.

Discontinuing clopidogrel prior to major surgery during the first 3 weeks after PCI predisposed to delayed stent thrombosis (Ong et al. 2005b, Spertus et al. 2006) and mortality rates that range from 30% (Ferrari et al. 2005) - 86% (Sharma et al. 2004). The timing of elective surgery is often dependent on the clinical circumstances in which clopidogrel has been prescribed. As previously mentioned, clopidogrel therapy is recommended for at least 4 weeks after placement of a BMS. The incidence of thrombotic complications and/or perioperative haemorrhage is extremely high in patients that discontinue clopidogrel prior to non-cardiac surgery requiring general anaesthesia (Kaluza et al. 2000, Wilson et al. 2003). Therefore, elective procedures for which there is significant risk of perioperative bleeding should be delayed until patients have completed an appropriate course of thienopyridine therapy. Two recent studies have emphasised the increased risk of stent thrombosis after non-cardiac surgery post DES insertion (Howard-Alpe et al. 2007, Brilakis et al. 2007). This risk is increased if surgery is performed early after stenting and particularly if dual antiplatelet therapy is discontinued.

Two additional large retrospective studies have also examined the incidence of major adverse cardiac events (MACE) in the perioperative period of non-cardiac surgery in patients with BMS and DES in relationship to the time from intracoronary stent placement (Nuttall et al. 2008, Sharma et al. 2004). Patients with BMS had a significantly lower risk of MACE as compared to patients with DES when non-cardiac surgery took place ≥ 30 days after stent placement (3.8% versus 10.4%) (Nuttall et al. 2008). On the other hand, patients with DES had a lower incidence of MACE as compared to patients with BMS when undergoing non-cardiac surgery ≥ 1 year after PCI (3.3% versus 6.0%) (Rabbitts et al. 2008). On univariate analysis, discontinuation of clopidogrel prior to non-cardiac surgery was a significant predictor for MACE. The authors conclude by suggesting that the lowest risk for MACE occurs after 1 year for DES and after 90 days for BMS.

Guidelines from the French Society of Anesthesiology and Intensive Care describe an algorithm for patients receiving clopidogrel and aspirin after insertion of a DES who require surgery (Collet et al. 2006). This multidisciplinary effort involves the surgeon and anaesthetist assessing the bleeding risk, the cardiologist evaluating the risk of stent thrombosis, and all three healthcare professional formulating an individual patient tailored management plan. It is noteworthy that full recovery of platelet function requires complete replacement of exposed platelets. However, adequate haemostasis does not require 100% of all circulating platelets to be functional. The CURE trial has demonstrated that clopidogrel therapy could be discontinued at least 5 days prior to coronary artery bypass graft (CABG) with no increased bleeding complications (Yusuf et al. 2001). Therefore, discontinuation at least 5 days preoperatively should permit adequate haemostasis prior to most surgical procedures (Gupta et al. 2012). In comparison, the American College of Chest Physicians suggest discontinuing the agent 7-10 days preoperatively and recommencing it 24 hours postoperatively or the following morning (Douketis et al. 2008, Douketis et al. 2012).

In patients who are receiving clopidogrel and are undergoing non-cardiac surgery, there are no randomised trials or prospective cohort studies that compare the clinical benefits and risks of continuing clopidogrel versus their temporary interruption. In particular, studies in patients undergoing abdominal or pelvic surgery are limited. Retrospective cohort studies have demonstrated increased rates of bleeding with perioperative continuation of clopidogrel (Sharma et al. 2004, Reddy and Vaitkus 2005). In addition, one prospective cohort study in patients who underwent bronchoscopy found significantly higher incidences of moderate or severe bleeding after biopsy in patients who received clopidogrel (61%) (Ernst et al. 2006).

If clopidogrel therapy is resumed with 75 mg/day, it takes five or more days to achieve maximal platelet function inhibition (Weber et al. 2001). Conversely, if therapy is resumed with a loading dose of 300 mg/day maximum platelet inhibition occurs within 2–15 hours after administration; however this increased dose is also associated with an increase in the risk of haemorrhage. Typically, resumption of a specific dose depends on a number of factors such as the perceived risk of thrombosis, the presence of a coronary stent, the type of stent implanted and the duration the stent has been implanted.

Platelet function assays are available to measure the antiplatelet activity of clopidogrel prior to surgery (Geiger et al. 2005). However, these methodologies are not well studied outside the percutaneous coronary intervention (PCI) setting (Steinhubl et al. 2001). Furthermore, the clinical significance of the assay results is uncertain as they have not been shown to identify patients at increased risk for perioperative bleeding (Geiger et al. 2005). Additional studies are needed to identify the potential of platelet function assays before their clinical applicability can be truly characterised.

7. PERIOPEREATIVE MANAGEMENT OF CLOPIDOGREL IN UROLOGICAL SURGERY

There are limited studies available for perioperative management of clopidogrel in urological patients. One prospective study assessed the safety for continuing clopidogrel therapy for transrectal ultrasound (TRUS) guided biopsy of the prostate in 13 patients on clopidogrel. Their findings suggest that discontinuation of the agent may not be necessary as only one patient develop bleeding during the postoperative period. Importantly, larger prospective studies will be required before this practice may be established routinely.

Another recent retrospective observational study using photoselective laser vaporisation of the prostate found no significant difference in blood loss between patients taking clopidogrel compared with a control group of patients (Ruszat et al. 2007, Sandhu et al. 2005). On the other hand it has also been demonstrated that clopidogrel therapy is associated with increased risk of haematoma formation in patients undergoing external shockwave lithotripsy (Knorr and Woodside 1990, Sare et al. 2002); however, no data is available for clopidogrel in patients undergoing major urological surgery such as nephrectomy, cystectomy or prostatectomy. Not surprisingly, one retrospective review of >1000 patients undergoing partial nephrectomy noted no difference in bleeding among patients taking clopidogrel when the agent was discontinued 10 days preoperatively (Kefer et al. 2009). Similar findings have also been noted with respect to clopidogrel and flexible ureterorenoscopy and holmium:YAG lithotripsy (Turna et al. 2008).

Results from other recent observational studies demonstrated a wide variation in the percentage of urologists that continue clopidogrel prior to specific urological procedures (Davis et al. 2011, NF Davis 2010).

Table 2. Percentage of consultant urologists that continue clopidogrel during the perioperative period for specific urological procedures (Davis NF 2010)

Procedure	Clopidogrel (%)
Circumcision (n=200)	13
TRUS + biopsy (n=198)	8
Cystoscopy + biopsy (n=193)	22
TURP (n=192)	2
TURBT (n=193)	3
Urethrotomy (n=193)	10
Diagnostic ureteroscopy (n=185)	50
Ureteroscopy+stone fragmentation (n=185)	19
Laparoscopic nephrectomy (n=160)	2
Radical cystectomy (n=154)	2
Open radical prostatectomy (n=150)	1

Furthermore, the aforementioned study also demonstrated significant variations in the number of days clopidogrel is routinely discontinued preoperatively and recommenced postoperatively among urological surgeons (Davis NF 2010).

As previously discussed; platelet function studies suggest that recovery of platelet function (sufficient for haemostasis) occurs within 5-7 days after discontinuing clopidogrel; however the majority of urological surgeons with Great Britain and Ireland discontinue the agent 7-9 days preoperatively (range 1 to >15 days) (Weber et al. 2001). Postoperatively, clopidogrel was most frequently recommenced after 1-3 days (range 1 to >15 days) which is consistent with studies that suggest recommencing the agent within 12-24 hours provided adequate intraoperative haemostasis is achieved (Douketis et al. 2012).

Table 3. Number of days that clopidogrel is discontinued before specific urological procedure according to urological surgeons (depicted as percentage) (Davis NF 2010)

Procedure	1-3 days (%)	4-6 days (%)	7-9 days (%)	10-12 days (%)	13-15 days (%)	>15 days (%)
Circumcision	9	18	39	20	14	0
TRUS + biopsy	7	13	50	16	14	0
Cystoscopy + biopsy	11	11	49	26	3	0
TURP	4	14	51	11	20	0
TURBT	4	15	52	19	10	0
Urethrotomy	7	16	52	20	4	1
Diagnostic ureteroscopy	9	18	46	27	0	0
Ureteroscopy+stone fragmentation	3	21	44	23	9	0
Laparoscopic nephrectomy	4	15	49	13	19	0
Radical cystectomy	2	14	46	18	20	0
Open radical prostatectomy	2	14	44	22	10	0

Table 4. Number of days that clopidogrel is recommenced after specific urological procedure according to urological surgeons (depicted as percentage) (Davis NF 2010)

Procedure	1-3 days (%)	4-6 days (%)	7-9 days (%)	10-12 days (%)	13-15 days (%)	>15 days (%)
Circumcision	38	11	49	0	2	0
TRUS + biopsy	41	7	49	1	2	0
Cystoscopy + biopsy	37	11	48	0	4	0
TURP	34	10	43	5	8	0
TURBT	32	12	45	5	6	0
Urethrotomy	39	8	48	2	3	0
Diagnostic ureteroscopy	39	11	50	0	0	0
Ureteroscopy + stone fragmentation	40	6	48	3	3	0
Laparoscopic nephrectomy	38	9	46	5	2	0
Radical cystectomy	29	15	44	5	7	0
Open radical prostatectomy	34	9	43	6	8	0

Table 5. Recommendations for perioperative clopidogrel management after initial dual antiplatelet therapy (1 month for BMS and 1 year for DES) is completed (Gupta et al. 2012)

Bleeding risk	Type of procedure	Preoperative modifications	Resuming clopidogrel
Low	Endoscopy (cystoscopy, ureteroscopy), laser lithotripsy, laser prostatectomy, urethral bulking procedures	Discontinue clopidogrel.	Recommence clopidogrel within 24 – 48 h postoperatively if no concern for bleeding
Moderate	TRUS, TURBT, ESWL, TURP, scrotal procedures, urinary sphincter placement, sling placements, female prolapse repair	Discontinue aspirin and clopidogrel therapy 5 – 7 days before procedure	Recommence dual antiplatelet therapy within 7 days of procedure if no concern for postoperative bleeding
High	Nephrectomy, cystectomy, prostatectomy, partial nephrectomy, penectomy, penile prosthesis placement	Discontinue dual antiplatelet therapy 10 days before procedure	Re-start antiplatelet therapy when no concern for active bleeding in coordination with cardiologist (7 – 10 days after no active bleeding)

One recent review developed a management strategy based on risk stratification for patients undergoing urological intervention on clopidogrel therapy after dual antiplatelet therapy. Their proposed guidelines are summarised in Table 5.

CONCLUSION

As the number of patients with coronary stents on clopidogrel therapy continues to increase, an evidence-based protocol for patients on antiplatelet therapy is imperative. For optimal outcomes it is clear that a multidisciplinary approach, including a cardiologist, surgeon, and anaesthetist are necessary for careful assessment of thrombotic and bleeding risks. Standardised perioperative guidelines based on risk-stratification should decrease the current variations in management protocols for clopidogrel among urological surgeons. The development of predefined urology-specific guidelines will almost inevitably improve the outcomes of patients on clopidogrel therapy undergoing urological surgery in the future.

REFERENCES

Akowuah, E., Shrivastava, V., Jamnadas, B., Hopkinson, D., Sarkar, P., Storey, R., Braidley, P. and Cooper, G. (2005). 'Comparison of two strategies for the management of antiplatelet therapy during urgent surgery', *Ann Thorac Surg*, *80*(1), 149-52.

Albaladejo, P., Marret, E., Piriou, V. and Samama, C. M. (2006). 'Perioperative management of antiplatelet agents in patients with coronary stents: recommendations of a French Task Force', *Br J Anaesth*, 97(4), 580-2.

Altman, R., Scazziota, A., M, D. E. L. H. and Gonzalez, C. (2006). 'Recombinant factor VIIa reverses the inhibitory effect of aspirin or aspirin plus clopidogrel on in vitro thrombin generation', *J Thromb Haemost*, *4*(9), 2022-7.

Angiolillo, D. J., Fernandez-Ortiz, A., Bernardo, E., Ramirez, C., Sabate, M., Jimenez-Quevedo, P., Hernandez, R., Moreno, R., Escaned, J., Alfonso, F., Banuelos, C., Costa, M. A., Bass, T. A. and Macaya, C. (2006). 'Clopidogrel withdrawal is associated with proinflammatory and prothrombotic effects in patients with diabetes and coronary artery disease', *Diabetes*, *55*(3), 780-4.

Arom, K. V. and Emery, R. W. (1994). 'Decreased postoperative drainage with addition of epsilon-aminocaproic acid before cardiopulmonary bypass', *Ann Thorac Surg*, *57*(5), 1108-12; discussion 1112-3.

Bavry, A. A. and Bhatt, D. L. (2008). 'Appropriate use of drug-eluting stents: balancing the reduction in restenosis with the concern of late thrombosis', *Lancet*, *371*(9630), 2134-43.

Bertrand, M. E., Rupprecht, H. J., Urban, P. and Gershlick, A. H. (2000). 'Double-blind study of the safety of clopidogrel with and without a loading dose in combination with aspirin compared with ticlopidine in combination with aspirin after coronary stenting : the clopidogrel aspirin stent international cooperative study (CLASSICS)', *Circulation*, *102*(6), 624-9.

Bhatt, D. L., Chew, D. P., Hirsch, A. T., Ringleb, P. A., Hacke, W. and Topol, E. J. (2001). 'Superiority of clopidogrel versus aspirin in patients with prior cardiac surgery', *Circulation*, *103*(3), 363-8.

Bhatt, D. L., Fox, K. A., Hacke, W., Berger, P. B., Black, H. R., Boden, W. E., Cacoub, P., Cohen, E. A., Creager, M. A., Easton, J. D., Flather, M. D., Haffner, S. M., Hamm, C. W., Hankey, G. J., Johnston, S. C., Mak, K. H., Mas, J. L., Montalescot, G., Pearson, T. A., Steg, P. G., Steinhubl, S. R., Weber, M. A., Brennan, D. M., Fabry-Ribaudo, L., Booth, J. and Topol, E. J. (2006). 'Clopidogrel and aspirin versus aspirin alone for the prevention of atherothrombotic events', *N Engl J Med*, *354*(16), 1706-17.

Bhatt, D. L., Marso, S. P., Hirsch, A. T., Ringleb, P. A., Hacke, W. and Topol, E. J. (2002). 'Amplified benefit of clopidogrel versus aspirin in patients with diabetes mellitus', *Am J Cardiol*, *90*(6), 625-8.

Biondi-Zoccai, G. G., Lotrionte, M., Agostoni, P., Abbate, A., Fusaro, M., Burzotta, F., Testa, L., Sheiban, I. and Sangiorgi, G. (2006). 'A systematic review and meta-analysis on the hazards of discontinuing or not adhering to aspirin among 50,279 patients at risk for coronary artery disease', *Eur Heart J*, *27*(22), 2667-74.

Brilakis, E. S., Banerjee, S. and Berger, P. B. (2007). 'Perioperative management of patients with coronary stents', *J Am Coll Cardiol*, *49*(22), 2145-50.

Burger, W., Chemnitius, J. M., Kneissl, G. D. and Rucker, G. (2005). 'Low-dose aspirin for secondary cardiovascular prevention - cardiovascular risks after its perioperative withdrawal versus bleeding risks with its continuation - review and meta-analysis', *J Intern Med*, *257*(5), 399-414.

Chassot, P. G., Delabays, A. and Spahn, D. R. (2007). 'Perioperative antiplatelet therapy: the case for continuing therapy in patients at risk of myocardial infarction', *Br J Anaesth*, *99*(3), 316-28.

Chesebro, J. H., Knatterud, G., Roberts, R., Borer, J., Cohen, L. S., Dalen, J., Dodge, H. T., Francis, C. K., Hillis, D., Ludbrook, P. and et al. (1987). 'Thrombolysis in Myocardial Infarction (TIMI). Trial, Phase I: A comparison between intravenous tissue plasminogen activator and intravenous streptokinase. Clinical findings through hospital discharge', *Circulation*, *76*(1), 142-54.

'Collaborative meta-analysis of randomised trials of antiplatelet therapy for prevention of death, myocardial infarction, and stroke in high risk patients', (2002). *BMJ*, *324*(7329), 71-86.

Collet, J. P., Montalescot, G., Le May, M., Borentain, M. and Gershlick, A. (2006). 'Percutaneous coronary intervention after fibrinolysis: a multiple meta-analyses approach according to the type of strategy', *J Am Coll Cardiol*, *48*(7), 1326-35.

Connor, S. E. and Wingate, J. P. (1999). 'Management of patients treated with aspirin or warfarin and evaluation of haemostasis prior to prostatic biopsy: a survey of current practice amongst radiologists and urologists', *Clin Radiol*, *54*(9), 598-603.

Davi, G. and Patrono, C. (2007). 'Platelet activation and atherothrombosis', *N Engl J Med*, *357*(24), 2482-94.

Davis, N. F., Fanning, D. M., McGuire, B. B., Carroll, G. T. and Flood, H. D. (2011). 'Perioperative management of chronic anticoagulation therapy in urological patients: a cross-sectional survey of practice', *Ir J Med Sci*, *180*(4), 823-8.

Davis NF, M. B., Flood HD (2010). 'Perioperative management of antithrombotic agents in urological surgery', *British Journal of Medical and Surgical Urology*, *4*(5), 187-196.

Douketis, J. D., Berger, P. B., Dunn, A. S., Jaffer, A. K., Spyropoulos, A. C., Becker, R. C. and Ansell, J. (2008). 'The perioperative management of antithrombotic therapy: American College of Chest Physicians Evidence-Based Clinical Practice Guidelines (8th Edition)', *Chest*, *133*(6 Suppl), 299S-339S.

Douketis, J. D., Spyropoulos, A. C., Spencer, F. A., Mayr, M., Jaffer, A. K., Eckman, M. H., Dunn, A. S. and Kunz, R. (2012). 'Perioperative management of antithrombotic therapy: Antithrombotic Therapy and Prevention of Thrombosis, 9th ed: American College of Chest Physicians

Evidence-Based Clinical Practice Guidelines', *Chest*, *141*(2 Suppl), e326S-50S.

Eagle, K. A., Berger, P. B., Calkins, H., Chaitman, B. R., Ewy, G. A., Fleischmann, K. E., Fleisher, L. A., Froehlich, J. B., Gusberg, R. J., Leppo, J. A., Ryan, T., Schlant, R. C., Winters, W. L., Jr., Gibbons, R. J., Antman, E. M., Alpert, J. S., Faxon, D. P., Fuster, V., Gregoratos, G., Jacobs, A. K., Hiratzka, L. F., Russell, R. O. and Smith, S. C., Jr. (2002). 'ACC/AHA guideline update for perioperative cardiovascular evaluation for noncardiac surgery---executive summary a report of the American College of Cardiology/American Heart Association Task Force on Practice Guidelines (Committee to Update the 1996 Guidelines on Perioperative Cardiovascular Evaluation for Noncardiac Surgery)', *Circulation*, *105*(10), 1257-67.

Eberli, D., Chassot, P. G., Sulser, T., Samama, C. M., Mantz, J., Delabays, A. and Spahn, D. R. (2010). 'Urological surgery and antiplatelet drugs after cardiac and cerebrovascular accidents', *J Urol*, *183*(6), 2128-36.

Eikelboom, J. W. (2006). 'The Outpatient Bleeding Risk Index predicted major bleeding in patients taking warfarin', *Evid Based Med*, *11*(4), 120.

Ernst, A., Eberhardt, R., Wahidi, M., Becker, H. D. and Herth, F. J. (2006). 'Effect of routine clopidogrel use on bleeding complications after transbronchial biopsy in humans', *Chest*, *129*(3), 734-7.

Ferrari, E., Benhamou, M., Cerboni, P. and Marcel, B. (2005). 'Coronary syndromes following aspirin withdrawal: a special risk for late stent thrombosis', *J Am Coll Cardiol*, *45*(3), 456-9.

Geiger, J., Teichmann, L., Grossmann, R., Aktas, B., Steigerwald, U., Walter, U. and Schinzel, R. (2005). 'Monitoring of clopidogrel action: comparison of methods', *Clin Chem*, *51*(6), 957-65.

Giannarini, G., Mogorovich, A., Valent, F., Morelli, G., De Maria, M., Manassero, F., Barbone, F. and Selli, C. (2007). 'Continuing or discontinuing low-dose aspirin before transrectal prostate biopsy: results of a prospective randomized trial', *Urology*, *70*(3), 501-5.

Grines, C. L., Bonow, R. O., Casey, D. E., Jr., Gardner, T. J., Lockhart, P. B., Moliterno, D. J., O'Gara, P. and Whitlow, P. (2007). 'Prevention of premature discontinuation of dual antiplatelet therapy in patients with coronary artery stents: a science advisory from the American Heart Association, American College of Cardiology, Society for Cardiovascular Angiography and Interventions, American College of Surgeons, and American Dental Association, with representation from the American College of Physicians', *Circulation*, *115*(6), 813-8.

Gupta, A. D., Streiff, M., Resar, J. and Schoenberg, M. (2012). 'Coronary stent management in elective genitourinary surgery', *BJU Int*, 110(4), 480-4.

Heit, J. A. (2001). 'Perioperative management of the chronically anticoagulated patient', *J Thromb Thrombolysis*, *12*(1), 81-7.

Howard-Alpe, G. M., de Bono, J., Hudsmith, L., Orr, W. P., Foex, P. and Sear, J. W. (2007). 'Coronary artery stents and non-cardiac surgery', *Br J Anaesth*, *98*(5), 560-74.

Iakovou, I., Schmidt, T., Bonizzoni, E., Ge, L., Sangiorgi, G. M., Stankovic, G., Airoldi, F., Chieffo, A., Montorfano, M., Carlino, M., Michev, I., Corvaja, N., Briguori, C., Gerckens, U., Grube, E. and Colombo, A. (2005). 'Incidence, predictors, and outcome of thrombosis after successful implantation of drug-eluting stents', *JAMA*, *293*(17), 2126-30.

"An international randomized trial comparing four thrombolytic strategies for acute myocardial infarction. The GUSTO investigators," (1993). *N Engl J Med*, *329*(10), 673-82.

Jeremias, A., Sylvia, B., Bridges, J., Kirtane, A. J., Bigelow, B., Pinto, D. S., Ho, K. K., Cohen, D. J., Garcia, L. A., Cutlip, D. E. and Carrozza, J. P., Jr. (2004). 'Stent thrombosis after successful sirolimus-eluting stent implantation', *Circulation*, *109*(16), 1930-2.

Kaiser, C., Brunner-La Rocca, H. P., Buser, P. T., Bonetti, P. O., Osswald, S., Linka, A., Bernheim, A., Zutter, A., Zellweger, M., Grize, L. and Pfisterer, M. E. (2005). 'Incremental cost-effectiveness of drug-eluting stents compared with a third-generation bare-metal stent in a real-world setting: randomised Basel Stent Kosten Effektivitats Trial (BASKET)', *Lancet*, *366*(9489), 921-9.

Kaluza, G. L., Joseph, J., Lee, J. R., Raizner, M. E. and Raizner, A. E. (2000). 'Catastrophic outcomes of noncardiac surgery soon after coronary stenting', *J Am Coll Cardiol*, *35*(5), 1288-94.

Kapoor, J. R. (2008). 'Platelet activation and atherothrombosis', *N Engl J Med*, *358*(15), 1638, author reply 1638-9.

Kastrati, A., Mehilli, J., Schuhlen, H., Dirschinger, J., Dotzer, F., ten Berg, J. M., Neumann, F. J., Bollwein, H., Volmer, C., Gawaz, M., Berger, P. B. and Schomig, A. (2004). 'A clinical trial of abciximab in elective percutaneous coronary intervention after pretreatment with clopidogrel', *N Engl J Med*, *350*(3), 232-8.

Kaushansky, K. (1998). 'Thrombopoietin', *N Engl J Med*, *339*(11), 746-54.

Kefer, J. C., Turna, B., Stein, R. J. and Desai, M. M. (2009). 'Safety and efficacy of percutaneous nephrostolithotomy in patients on anticoagulant therapy', *J Urol*, *181*(1), 144-8.

Knorr, P. A. and Woodside, J. R. (1990). 'Large perirenal hematoma after extracorporeal shock-wave lithotripsy', *Urology*, *35*(2), 151-3.

Kuchulakanti, P. K., Chu, W. W., Torguson, R., Ohlmann, P., Rha, S. W., Clavijo, L. C., Kim, S. W., Bui, A., Gevorkian, N., Xue, Z., Smith, K., Fournadjieva, J., Suddath, W. O., Satler, L. F., Pichard, A. D., Kent, K. M. and Waksman, R. (2006). 'Correlates and long-term outcomes of angiographically proven stent thrombosis with sirolimus- and paclitaxel-eluting stents', *Circulation*, *113*(8), 1108-13.

Lagerqvist, B., James, S. K., Stenestrand, U., Lindback, J., Nilsson, T. and Wallentin, L. (2007). 'Long-term outcomes with drug-eluting stents versus bare-metal stents in Sweden', *N Engl J Med*, *356*(10), 1009-19.

Levi, M., Cromheecke, M. E., de Jonge, E., Prins, M. H., de Mol, B. J., Briet, E. and Buller, H. R. (1999). 'Pharmacological strategies to decrease excessive blood loss in cardiac surgery: a meta-analysis of clinically relevant endpoints', *Lancet*, *354*(9194), 1940-7.

Levy, J. (1960). '[Pharmacological comparisons of the medicinal substances favoring or inhibiting the synthesis, mobilization and preservation of the biogenic amines of the brain (catecholamines and indolamines)]', *Therapie*, *15*, 1279-94.

Lindvall, G., Sartipy, U. and van der Linden, J. (2005). 'Aprotinin reduces bleeding and blood product use in patients treated with clopidogrel before coronary artery bypass grafting', *Ann Thorac Surg*, *80*(3), 922-7.

McFadden, E. P., Stabile, E., Regar, E., Cheneau, E., Ong, A. T., Kinnaird, T., Suddath, W. O., Weissman, N. J., Torguson, R., Kent, K. M., Pichard, A. D., Satler, L. F., Waksman, R. and Serruys, P. W. (2004). 'Late thrombosis in drug-eluting coronary stents after discontinuation of antiplatelet therapy', *Lancet*, *364*(9444), 1519-21.

Mehta, S. R., Yusuf, S., Peters, R. J., Bertrand, M. E., Lewis, B. S., Natarajan, M. K., Malmberg, K., Rupprecht, H., Zhao, F., Chrolavicius, S., Copland, I. and Fox, K. A. (2001). 'Effects of pretreatment with clopidogrel and aspirin followed by long-term therapy in patients undergoing percutaneous coronary intervention: the PCI-CURE study', *Lancet*, *358*(9281), 527-33.

Moscucci, M., Fox, K. A., Cannon, C. P., Klein, W., Lopez-Sendon, J., Montalescot, G., White, K. and Goldberg, R. J. (2003). 'Predictors of major bleeding in acute coronary syndromes: the Global Registry of Acute Coronary Events (GRACE)', *Eur Heart J*, *24*(20), 1815-23.

Muller, I., Seyfarth, M., Rudiger, S., Wolf, B., Pogatsa-Murray, G., Schomig, A. and Gawaz, M. (2001). 'Effect of a high loading dose of clopidogrel on platelet function in patients undergoing coronary stent placement', *Heart*, *85*(1), 92-3.

Nakazawa, G., Finn, A. V., Joner, M., Ladich, E., Kutys, R., Mont, E. K., Gold, H. K., Burke, A. P., Kolodgie, F. D. and Virmani, R. (2008). 'Delayed arterial healing and increased late stent thrombosis at culprit sites after drug-eluting stent placement for acute myocardial infarction patients: an autopsy study', *Circulation*, *118*(11), 1138-45.

NF Davis, B. M., HD Flood (2010). 'Perioperative management of antithrombotic agents in urological surgery', *British Journal of Medical and Surgical Urology*, *4*(5), 187-196.

Nuttall, G. A., Brown, M. J., Stombaugh, J. W., Michon, P. B., Hathaway, M. F., Lindeen, K. C., Hanson, A. C., Schroeder, D. R., Oliver, W. C., Holmes, D. R. and Rihal, C. S. (2008). 'Time and cardiac risk of surgery after bare-metal stent percutaneous coronary intervention', *Anesthesiology*, *109*(4), 588-95.

O'Riordan, J. M., Margey, R. J., Blake, G. and O'Connell, P. R. (2009). 'Antiplatelet agents in the perioperative period', *Arch Surg*, *144*(1), 69-76; discussion 76.

Ong, A. T., Hoye, A., Aoki, J., van Mieghem, C. A., Rodriguez Granillo, G. A., Sonnenschein, K., Regar, E., McFadden, E. P., Sianos, G., van der Giessen, W. J., de Jaegere, P. P., de Feyter, P., van Domburg, R. T. and Serruys, P. W. (2005a). 'Thirty-day incidence and six-month clinical outcome of thrombotic stent occlusion after bare-metal, sirolimus, or paclitaxel stent implantation', *J Am Coll Cardiol*, *45*(6), 947-53.

Ong, A. T., McFadden, E. P., Regar, E., de Jaegere, P. P., van Domburg, R. T. and Serruys, P. W. (2005b). 'Late angiographic stent thrombosis (LAST). events with drug-eluting stents', *J Am Coll Cardiol*, *45*(12), 2088-92.

Park, D. W., Park, S. W., Park, K. H., Lee, B. K., Kim, Y. H., Lee, C. W., Hong, M. K., Kim, J. J. and Park, S. J. (2006). 'Frequency of and risk factors for stent thrombosis after drug-eluting stent implantation during long-term follow-up', *Am J Cardiol*, *98*(3), 352-6.

Pfisterer, M., Brunner-La Rocca, H. P., Buser, P. T., Rickenbacher, P., Hunziker, P., Mueller, C., Jeger, R., Bader, F., Osswald, S. and Kaiser, C. (2006). 'Late clinical events after clopidogrel discontinuation may limit the benefit of drug-eluting stents: an observational study of drug-eluting versus bare-metal stents', *J Am Coll Cardiol*, *48*(12), 2584-91.

Rabbitts, J. A., Nuttall, G. A., Brown, M. J., Hanson, A. C., Oliver, W. C., Holmes, D. R. and Rihal, C. S. (2008). 'Cardiac risk of noncardiac surgery after percutaneous coronary intervention with drug-eluting stents', *Anesthesiology*, *109*(4), 596-604.

Rao, S. V., O'Grady, K., Pieper, K. S., Granger, C. B., Newby, L. K., Van de Werf, F., Mahaffey, K. W., Califf, R. M. and Harrington, R. A. (2005). 'Impact of bleeding severity on clinical outcomes among patients with acute coronary syndromes', *Am J Cardiol*, *96*(9), 1200-6.

Reddy, P. R. and Vaitkus, P. T. (2005). 'Risks of noncardiac surgery after coronary stenting', *Am J Cardiol*, *95*(6), 755-7.

Ringleb, P. A., Bhatt, D. L., Hirsch, A. T., Topol, E. J. and Hacke, W. (2004). 'Benefit of clopidogrel over aspirin is amplified in patients with a history of ischemic events', *Stroke*, *35*(2), 528-32.

Ruszat, R., Wyler, S., Forster, T., Reich, O., Stief, C. G., Gasser, T. C., Sulser, T. and Bachmann, A. (2007). 'Safety and effectiveness of photoselective vaporization of the prostate (PVP). in patients on ongoing oral anticoagulation', *Eur Urol*, *51*(4), 1031-8; discussion 1038-41.

Sandhu, J. S., Ng, C. K., Gonzalez, R. R., Kaplan, S. A. and Te, A. E. (2005). 'Photoselective laser vaporization prostatectomy in men receiving anticoagulants', *J Endourol*, *19*(10), 1196-8.

Sare, G. M., Lloyd, F. R. and Stower, M. J. (2002). 'Life-threatening haemorrhage after extracorporeal shockwave lithotripsy in a patient taking clopidogrel', *BJU Int*, *90*(4), 469.

Schulman, S. and Kearon, C. (2005). 'Definition of major bleeding in clinical investigations of antihemostatic medicinal products in non-surgical patients', *J Thromb Haemost*, *3*(4), 692-4.

Serruys, P. W., Kutryk, M. J. and Ong, A. T. (2006). 'Coronary-artery stents', *N Engl J Med*, *354*(5), 483-95.

Sharma, A. K., Ajani, A. E., Hamwi, S. M., Maniar, P., Lakhani, S. V., Waksman, R. and Lindsay, J. (2004). 'Major noncardiac surgery following coronary stenting: when is it safe to operate?', *Catheter Cardiovasc Interv*, *63*(2), 141-5.

Silber, S., Albertsson, P., Aviles, F. F., Camici, P. G., Colombo, A., Hamm, C., Jorgensen, E., Marco, J., Nordrehaug, J. E., Ruzyllo, W., Urban, P., Stone, G. W. and Wijns, W. (2005). 'Guidelines for percutaneous coronary interventions. The Task Force for Percutaneous Coronary Interventions of the European Society of Cardiology', *Eur Heart J*, *26*(8), 804-47.

Smith, S. C., Jr., Allen, J., Blair, S. N., Bonow, R. O., Brass, L. M., Fonarow, G. C., Grundy, S. M., Hiratzka, L., Jones, D., Krumholz, H. M., Mosca, L., Pasternak, R. C., Pearson, T., Pfeffer, M. A. and Taubert, K. A. (2006a). 'AHA/ACC guidelines for secondary prevention for patients with coronary and other atherosclerotic vascular disease: 2006 update: endorsed by the National Heart, Lung, and Blood Institute', *Circulation, 113*(19), 2363-72.

Smith, S. C., Jr., Feldman, T. E., Hirshfeld, J. W., Jr., Jacobs, A. K., Kern, M. J., King, S. B., 3rd, Morrison, D. A., O'Neill, W. W., Schaff, H. V., Whitlow, P. L., Williams, D. O., Antman, E. M., Adams, C. D., Anderson, J. L., Faxon, D. P., Fuster, V., Halperin, J. L., Hiratzka, L. F., Hunt, S. A., Nishimura, R., Ornato, J. P., Page, R. L. and Riegel, B. (2006b). 'ACC/AHA/SCAI 2005 Guideline Update for Percutaneous Coronary Intervention--summary article: a report of the American College of Cardiology/American Heart Association Task Force on Practice Guidelines (ACC/AHA/SCAI Writing Committee to Update the 2001 Guidelines for Percutaneous Coronary Intervention)', *Circulation, 113*(1), 156-75.

Spertus, J. A., Kettelkamp, R., Vance, C., Decker, C., Jones, P. G., Rumsfeld, J. S., Messenger, J. C., Khanal, S., Peterson, E. D., Bach, R. G., Krumholz, H. M. and Cohen, D. J. (2006). 'Prevalence, predictors, and outcomes of premature discontinuation of thienopyridine therapy after drug-eluting stent placement: results from the PREMIER registry', *Circulation, 113*(24), 2803-9.

Steinhubl, S. R., Berger, P. B., Mann, J. T., 3rd, Fry, E. T., DeLago, A., Wilmer, C. and Topol, E. J. (2002). 'Early and sustained dual oral antiplatelet therapy following percutaneous coronary intervention: a randomized controlled trial', *JAMA, 288*(19), 2411-20.

Steinhubl, S. R., Talley, J. D., Braden, G. A., Tcheng, J. E., Casterella, P. J., Moliterno, D. J., Navetta, F. I., Berger, P. B., Popma, J. J., Dangas, G., Gallo, R., Sane, D. C., Saucedo, J. F., Jia, G., Lincoff, A. M., Theroux, P., Holmes, D. R., Teirstein, P. S. and Kereiakes, D. J. (2001). 'Point-of-care measured platelet inhibition correlates with a reduced risk of an adverse cardiac event after percutaneous coronary intervention: results of the GOLD (AU-Assessing Ultegra). multicenter study', *Circulation, 103*(21), 2572-8.

Stettler, C., Wandel, S., Allemann, S., Kastrati, A., Morice, M. C., Schomig, A., Pfisterer, M. E., Stone, G. W., Leon, M. B., de Lezo, J. S., Goy, J. J., Park, S. J., Sabate, M., Suttorp, M. J., Kelbaek, H., Spaulding, C., Menichelli, M., Vermeersch, P., Dirksen, M. T., Cervinka, P., Petronio, A. S., Nordmann, A. J., Diem, P., Meier, B., Zwahlen, M., Reichenbach, S., Trelle, S., Windecker, S. and Juni, P. (2007). 'Outcomes associated with drug-eluting and bare-metal stents: a collaborative network meta-analysis', *Lancet*, *370*(9591), 937-48.

Turna, B., Stein, R. J., Smaldone, M. C., Santos, B. R., Kefer, J. C., Jackman, S. V., Averch, T. D. and Desai, M. M. (2008). 'Safety and efficacy of flexible ureterorenoscopy and holmium:YAG lithotripsy for intrarenal stones in anticoagulated cases', *J Urol*, *179*(4), 1415-9.

Urban, P., Gershlick, A. H., Guagliumi, G., Guyon, P., Lotan, C., Schofer, J., Seth, A., Sousa, J. E., Wijns, W., Berge, C., Deme, M. and Stoll, H. P. (2006). 'Safety of coronary sirolimus-eluting stents in daily clinical practice: one-year follow-up of the e-Cypher registry', *Circulation*, *113*(11), 1434-41.

van der Linden, J., Lindvall, G. and Sartipy, U. (2005). 'Aprotinin decreases postoperative bleeding and number of transfusions in patients on clopidogrel undergoing coronary artery bypass graft surgery: a double-blind, placebo-controlled, randomized clinical trial', *Circulation*, *112*(9 Suppl), I276-80.

Vilahur, G., Choi, B. G., Zafar, M. U., Viles-Gonzalez, J. F., Vorchheimer, D. A., Fuster, V. and Badimon, J. J. (2007). 'Normalization of platelet reactivity in clopidogrel-treated subjects', *J Thromb Haemost*, *5*(1), 82-90.

von Heymann, C., Schoenfeld, H., Sander, M., Ziemer, S., Grubitzsch, H. and Spies, C. (2005). 'Clopidogrel-related refractory bleeding after coronary artery bypass graft surgery: a rationale for the use of coagulation factor concentrates?', *Heart Surg Forum*, *8*(1), E39-41.

Weber, A. A., Braun, M., Hohlfeld, T., Schwippert, B., Tschope, D. and Schror, K. (2001). 'Recovery of platelet function after discontinuation of clopidogrel treatment in healthy volunteers', *Br J Clin Pharmacol*, *52*(3), 333-6.

Williams, D. O., Abbott, J. D. and Kip, K. E. (2006). 'Outcomes of 6906 patients undergoing percutaneous coronary intervention in the era of drug-eluting stents: report of the DEScover Registry', *Circulation*, *114*(20), 2154-62.

Wilson, S. H., Fasseas, P., Orford, J. L., Lennon, R. J., Horlocker, T., Charnoff, N. E., Melby, S. and Berger, P. B. (2003). 'Clinical outcome of patients undergoing non-cardiac surgery in the two months following coronary stenting', *J Am Coll Cardiol*, *42*(2), 234-40.

Yusuf, S., Zhao, F., Mehta, S. R., Chrolavicius, S., Tognoni, G. and Fox, K. K. (2001). 'Effects of clopidogrel in addition to aspirin in patients with acute coronary syndromes without ST-segment elevation', *N Engl J Med*, *345*(7), 494-502.

In: Clopidogrel
Editors: J. P. Alesci and A. Victorino

ISBN: 978-1-62948-336-8
© 2014 Nova Science Publishers, Inc.

Chapter 8

PLATELET FUNCTION TESTING TO GUIDE THERAPY IN POOR RESPONDERS TO CLOPIDOGREL

Sattar Gojraty and Dmitriy N. Feldman*
Division of Cardiology, Weill Cornell Medical College,
New York Presbyterian Hospital, New York, NY, US

ABSTRACT

Dual oral antiplatelet therapy with aspirin and clopidogrel is the cornerstone of current therapy in patients with acute coronary syndromes and in patients undergoing percutaneous coronary intervention (PCI). Responsiveness to clopidogrel is not uniform and is subject to considerable interindividual variability. Furthermore, there are recent data that poor response to clopidogrel, or "high on-treatment platelet reactivity" (HPR), may be associated with the occurrence of ischemic events post-PCI. A variety of platelet function testing methods are currently available for evaluating platelet inhibition to clopidogrel, particularly in post-PCI patients, in order to determine and potentially reduce the individual risk for ischemic events. Platelet function testing offers the potential to individually tailor antiplatelet therapy.

* Corresponding author: Dmitriy N. Feldman, MD; Assistant Professor of Medicine, Weill Cornell Medical College, New York Presbyterian Hospital, Department of Medicine, Greenberg Division of Cardiology, 520 East 70th Street, Starr-4 Pavilion, New York, NY 10021. Phone: (212) 746-4644; Fax: (212) 746-8295; E-mail: dnf9001@med.cornell.edu.

Whether a personalized approach to intensified platelet inhibition therapy can be beneficial in higher risk patients remains to be determined and will require further prospective investigation. We will review in this chapter the impact of clopidogrel responsiveness on clinical outcomes and personalized antiplatelet strategies to improve clopidogrel responsiveness.

INTRODUCTION

Clopidogrel is a pro-drug in the thienopyridine class that is absorbed intestinally and transformed via hepatic activation by cytochrome P450 enzymes. The activated metabolite then binds and irreversibly inhibits the $P2Y_{12}$ subtype of the adenosine diphosphate (ADP) receptor by forming a disulfide bridge with the $P2Y_{12}$ ADP receptor. The activated G protein-coupled $P2Y_{12}$ receptor has downstream effects that eventually lead to ADP granules release and potentiate platelet aggregation.

Despite the wide use of clopidogrel in numerous clinical settings, variable platelet inhibitory response among patients taking clopidogrel has been described [1]. The CYP2C19 enzyme, perhaps the most clinically relevant constituent of the cytochrome P450 enzymes for clopidogrel metabolism, has been shown to significantly affect the individual response to clopidogrel [2, 3]. CYP2C19 can be affected by common genetic polymorphisms [4] leading to loss-of-function genetic variants that reduce its catalytic activity, resulting in reduced levels of active clopidogrel metabolite [5].

Patients with lower plasma concentrations of clopidogrel's active metabolite have been shown to have lower levels of inhibition of platelet aggregation [6]. In the GIFT study, a single nucleotide polymorphism was shown to be associated with reduced platelet inhibition in patients given clopidogrel after percutaneous coronary intervention [1]. Carriers of two loss-of-function CYP219 alleles were at even greater risk for high residual platelet reactivity on clopidogrel.

The metabolism of clopidogrel is affected by numerous other disease states and drugs. Cigarette smoking, for example, was found to have a dose-response effect on residual platelet reactivity to clopidogrel in diabetic patients, with heavier smokers having lower rates of high on-treatment platelet reactivity [7]. This is thought to be due to cigarette smoking being an inducer of CYP1A2, a hepatic enzyme involved in clopidogrel metabolism [7].

The presence of diabetes mellitus itself has also been associated with high residual platelet reactivity in patients receiving clopidogrel [8] along with several commonly used drugs including nitrates, statins, proton pump inhibitors, and calcium channel blockers [8, 9]. Additionally, gender and racial differences have been shown to have an effect on residual platelet reactivity in patients taking clopidogrel [8].

Given the large number of variables that can affect the degree of platelet inhibition by clopidogrel, platelet function testing has been an area of both clinical and commercial interest in the past several years. Using platelet function testing, clinicians can quantitatively assess the response to antiplatelet agents like clopidogrel, potentially allowing them to individualize antiplatelet therapy. Specifically, there has been substantial clinical interest in applying platelet function testing to patients undergoing coronary stent implantation.

ASSAYS USED FOR PLATELET FUNCTION TESTING

There are numerous commercially available assays for in-vitro testing of platelet function, each of which has its own strengths, weaknesses, and test characteristics. Multiple signaling pathways exist in platelet activation, but the majority of commercially available assays concentrate on the $P2Y_{12}$ receptor and its immediate downstream effects. Once this receptor binds to ADP, it activates a secondary messenger system that inhibits adenylyl cyclase, lowering intracellular levels of cyclic adenosine monophosphate (cAMP). Lower levels of cAMP, in turn, decrease the phosphorylation of vasodilator-stimulated phosphoprotein (VASP). The majority of platelet function assays, including light transmittance aggregometry [LTA] [10], multiple electrode aggregometry [11], Platelet Works [12], and VerifyNow $P2Y_{12}$ [13] artificially activate platelets using ADP to measure the degree of $P2Y_{12}$ receptor inhibition by ADP antagonists. The VASP assay instead uses flow cytometry to measure the phosphorylation status of VASP protein. The concentration of phosphorylated VASP protein correlates to platelet inhibition at the level of the $P2Y_{12}$ receptor [14]. A Comparison study investigated the ability of four major platelet function assays to identify clopidogrel-treated patients and inter-test variability [15]. The study evaluated 116 patients with stable coronary artery disease requiring diagnostic angiography, using blood samples that were obtained before and after clopidogrel initiation. The blood samples were tested for in-vitro platelet function using light transmission aggregometry (LTA), whole-blood aggregometry, VerifyNow P2Y12, and PFA-100. Agreement between assays to identify patients with insufficient inhibition of platelet aggregation by clopidogrel was low. The findings of this study emphasize that platelet function tests are highly test-specific and platelet function assays should not be considered interchangeable.

The Ability of Platelet Function Testing to Predict Clinical Response

High platelet reactivity in the setting of clopidogrel use has been shown in several studies to correlate with adverse clinical outcomes. A meta-analysis published in 2011 combined data from patients undergoing PCI who had their platelet reactivity tested using the VerifyNow $P2Y_{12}$ assay [16]. This meta-analysis examined 3,059 patients, separated into four quartiles of on-treatment $P2Y_{12}$ reactivity unit (PRU) values. The authors concluded that patients in the highest quartile had a hazard ratio (HR) of 2.62 for risk of death, myocardial infarction (MI), or stent thrombosis (95% CI: 1.78 to 3.87; $p < 0.001$). The risk then decreased step-wise between the highest and lowest quartiles (quartile III HR=1.82, $p = 0.005$; quartile II HR=1.13, $p = 0.60$; quartile I reference).

The relationship between platelet function testing and outcomes was also explored in a small population of patients experiencing ST-elevation myocardial infarction (STEMI) [17]. 60 consecutive patients who underwent primary angioplasty with stenting for acute STEMI were arranged into quartiles based on their percentage reduction of ADP-induced platelet aggregation. The patients in the highest quartile of clopidogrel resistance had a 40% incidence of cardiovascular events, compared with an incidence of 2.2% in patients in the lower three quartiles at 6-months.

GRAVITAS trial was a large, multicenter, double blind, randomized trial of platelet function testing in patients undergoing PCI [18]. The study compared two treatment strategies in patients with high on-treatment platelet reactivity (OTR) after percutaneous coronary intervention (PRU $\geq$230 by VerifyNow $P2Y_{12}$ platelet function test). A time-dependent analysis of the GRAVITAS study found that regardless of the treatment strategy that was used, lower OTR values were significantly associated with a lower risk of the combined endpoint: cardiovascular death, myocardial infarction, and stent thrombosis [19].

More recently, ADAPT-DES was a prospective, largest multicenter registry study that examined platelet reactivity in patients after drug-eluting stent (DES) implantation [20]. 8,583 eligible patients who were taking aspirin and clopidogrel had platelet reactivity evaluated using the Verify Now $P2Y_{12}$ platelet function test. Authors found that high platelet reactivity on clopidogrel was strongly related to stent thrombosis (HR 2.49, p=0.001) and myocardial infarction (HR 1.42, p=0.01), but was not related to mortality (HR 1.20, p=0.30) at 1 year.

These studies strongly suggest that platelet function testing can be valuable in identifying patients that are at high risk for coronary events post-PCI.

Value of Monitoring Platelet Function Pre- and Post-PCI

The first randomized trial to study the clinical impact of adjusting clopidogrel loading doses in patients undergoing PCI using platelet function testing was published in 2008 [21]. Authors used vasodilator-stimulated phosphoprotein phosphorylation (VASP) to quantify platelet inhibition by clopidogrel. 162 patients with VASP index > 50 after a 600-mg loading dose of clopidogrel were randomized into two groups prior to PCI, a VASP-guided therapy group and a control group. In the VASP-guided therapy group, patients received up to three additional doses of 600-mg of clopidogrel in 24-hour increments until their VASP index was less than 50 or they had received the maximum allotted three additional doses of clopidogrel. Patients were monitored for 1 month after PCI for any major adverse cardiovascular events (MACE), which included cardiovascular death, angiographically-confirmed stent thrombosis, recurrent acute coronary syndrome and recurrent revascularization (either coronary angioplasty or bypass surgery). In the VASP-guided therapy group, the additional clopidogrel doses reduced the VASP index to less than 50 in 86% of patients, the majority of which required one additional dose of clopidogrel. In the VASP-guided group, there were significantly fewer MACE events as compared to the control group (0% vs. 10%; p = 0.007). Moreover, there was no significant difference in major and minor bleeding between the VASP-guided group and the control group (5% vs. 4%; p = ns).

Using a much larger cohort of patients, the ARCTIC trial studied the benefit of monitoring platelet function prior to PCI in 2,440 patients who were undergoing coronary stenting [22]. Patients were randomized to a strategy of platelet function monitoring with intervention versus usual care without monitoring. The subset of patients that had high on-treatment platelet reactivity were given a glycoprotein IIb/IIIa inhibitor during PCI and an additional clopidogrel load (600-mg) or prasugrel, along with high-dose clopidogrel (150-mg daily) or prasugrel (10-mg daily) maintenance therapy. Patients were monitored for the primary endpoint, which was a composite of death, myocardial infarction, stent thrombosis, stroke, or urgent revascularization at one year. A large proportion of patients, 34.5%, were found to have high platelet reactivity in the setting of clopidogrel use. However, the primary endpoint occurred at similar rates between the platelet function monitoring group and the usual care group without platelet function testing (34.6% vs. 31.1%, p=0.10). The ARCTIC trial showed that platelet monitoring prior to and after PCI and adjusting treatment using either high-dose clopidogrel or prasugrel did not change outcomes at 1 year. ARCTIC-2 will evaluate a second randomization occurring one year after the first randomization to determine the effect of continuation versus interruption of clopidogrel therapy.

Routine monitoring of patients post-PCI was studied in the GRAVITAS trial [18]. Patients undergoing drug-eluting stent placement were tested using the VerifyNow assay, and the subset of patients with high on-treatment platelet reactivity (defined as 230 PRU or higher) were eligible for the trial. These patients were randomized into a high-dose clopidogrel arm (600-mg initial dose, 150-mg daily thereafter) or received standard of care, considered to be no additional loading dose with clopidogrel 75-mg daily for 6 months. The primary endpoint was death from cardiovascular causes, nonfatal MI, or stent thrombosis at 6 months. At 30-day follow-up, the patients in the high-dose group had a statistically significant reduction in the rate of high on-treatment platelet reactivity as compared to the standard-dose group. In addition, there was no increase in severe or moderate bleeding with the high-dose regimen. However, despite having lower rates of high on-treatment platelet reactivity, patients in the high-dose clopidogrel group experienced the same frequency of events as the patients in the standard-dose group (2.3% for both groups).

Two other smaller trials examined alternative treatment agents to clopidogrel in patients who were poor responders to clopidogrel. The 3T2R trial studied the use of tirofiban in 263 poor responders to aspirin and/or clopidogrel [23]. Patients undergoing elective coronary angioplasty were randomly assigned to receive either tirofiban or placebo on top of standard aspirin and clopidogrel therapy. The authors concluded that intensified platelet inhibition with tirofiban lowers the incidence of myocardial infarction after elective coronary intervention (20.4% tirofiban versus 35.1% placebo). The rate of major adverse cardiovascular events within 30 days in the tirofiban group also was reduced (3.8% versus 10.7%; p=0.031). TRIGGER-PCI trial intended to study patients with PRU > 208 by VerifyNow who were receiving a DES for stable coronary artery disease [24]. Patients with HPR were randomly assigned to receive prasugrel versus clopidogrel. The study was terminated early due to a lower rate than expected of adverse events of cardiac death or myocardial infarction.

Society Guidelines

The 2011 ACCF/AHA/SCAI Guidelines for Percutaneous Coronary Intervention recommend that platelet function testing may be considered in patients at high risk for poor clinical outcomes (Class IIb, Level of evidence C) [25]. Furthermore, in patients treated with clopidogrel with high platelet reactivity, alternative agents, such as prasugrel or ticagrelor, might be considered (Class IIb, Level of evidence C). The guidelines recommend against the routine use of platelet function testing to screen patients treated with clopidogrel who are undergoing PCI (Class III, Level of evidence C).

The 2012 ACCF/AHA Focused Update of the Guideline for the Management of Patients With Unstable Angina/Non-ST-Elevation Myocardial Infarction states that platelet function testing in patients with UA/NSTEMI may be considered if results of testing may alter further management (Class IIb, Level of evidence C) [26].

Conclusion

The assessment of platelet function inhibition by clopidogrel is highly heterogeneous and test-specific. Platelet function tests can identify patients with high on-treatment platelet reactivity and provide important prognostic information post-PCI. Given the heterogeneity of platelet function tests, each assay should be studied independently and results should not be considered interchangeable. Currently, given negative results of GRAVITAS, TRIGGER PCI and ARCTIC studies, routine platelet function testing and adjusting antiplatelet therapy based on the results of such testing in patients with stable coronary artery disease cannot be recommended. Further studies are needed to evaluate in which patients and clinical scenarios platelet function testing may be appropriate.

Conflict of Interest Disclosures

Dr. Feldman serves as a consultant/ speaker for Eli Lilly, Daiichi-Sankyo, The Medicines Company, Pfizer, and Bristol-Myers Squibb.

References

[1] Price, M. J., Murray, S. S., Angiolillo, D. J., Lillie, E., Smith, E. N., Tisch, R. L., Schork, N. J., Teirstein, P. S., Topol, E. J.; GIFT Investigators. Influence of genetic polymorphisms on the effect of high- and standard-dose clopidogrel after percutaneous coronary intervention: the GIFT (Genotype Information and Functional Testing) study. *J. Am. Coll. Cardiol.* 2012 May 29;59(22):1928-37.

[2] Kazui, M., Nishiya, Y., Ishizuka, T., Hagihara, K., Farid, N. A., Okazaki, O., Ikeda, T., Kurihara, A. Identification of the human cytochrome P450 enzymes involved in the two oxidative steps in the bioactivation of clopidogrel to its pharmacologically active metabolite. *Drug Metab. Dispos.* 2010 Jan;38(1):92-9.

[3] Shuldiner, A. R., O'Connell, J. R., Bliden, K. P., Gandhi, A., Ryan, K., Horenstein, R. B., Damcott, C. M., Pakyz, R., Tantry, U. S., Gibson, Q., Pollin, T. I., Post, W., Parsa, A., Mitchell, B. D., Faraday, N., Herzog, W., Gurbel, P. A. Association of cytochrome P450 2C19 genotype with the antiplatelet effect and clinical efficacy of clopidogrel therapy. *JAMA.* 2009 Aug. 26;302(8):849-57.

[4] Price, M. J., Tantry, U. S., Gurbel, P. A. The influence of CYP2C19 polymorphisms on the pharmacokinetics, pharmacodynamics, and clinical effectiveness of P2Y(12) inhibitors. *Rev. Cardiovasc. Med.* 2011; 12(1):1-12.

[5] Brandt, J. T., Close, S. L., Iturria, S. J., Payne, C. D., Farid, N. A., Ernest, C. S., et al. Common polymorphisms of CYP2C19 and CYP2C9 affect the pharmacokinetic and pharmacodynamic response to clopidogrel but not prasugrel. *J. Thromb. Haemost.* 2007 Dec;5(12): 2429-36.

[6] Brandt, J. T., Payne, C. D., Wiviott, S. D., Weerakkody, G., Farid, N. A., Small, D. S., Jakubowski, J. A., Naganuma, H., Winters, K. J. A comparison of prasugrel and clopidogrel loading doses on platelet function: magnitude of platelet inhibition is related to active metabolite formation. *Am. Heart J.* 2007 Jan;153(1):66.e9-16.

[7] Ueno, M., Ferreiro, J. L., Desai, B., Tomasello, S. D., Tello-Montoliu, A., Capodanno, D., Capranzano, P., Kodali, M., Dharmashankar, K., Charlton, R. K., Bass, T. A., Angiolillo, D. J. Cigarette smoking is associated with a dose-response effect in clopidogrel-treated patients with diabetes mellitus and coronary artery disease: results of a pharmacodynamic study. *JACC Cardiovasc. Interv.* 2012 Mar;5(3):293-300.

[8] Price, M. J., Nayak, K. R., Barker, C. M., Kandzari, D. E., Teirstein, P. S. Predictors of heightened platelet reactivity despite dual-antiplatelet therapy in patients undergoing percutaneous coronary intervention. *Am. J. Cardiol.* 2009 May 15;103(10):1339-43.

[9] Siller-Matula, J. M., Lang, I., Christ, G., Jilma, B. Calcium-channel blockers reduce the antiplatelet effect of clopidogrel. *J. Am. Coll. Cardiol.* 2008 Nov. 4;52(19):1557-63.

[10] Born, G. Aggregation of blood platelets by adenosine diphosphate and its reversal. *Nature*. 1962 Jun. 9;194:927-9.

[11] Toth, O., Calatzis, A., Penz, S., Losonczy, H., Siess, W. Multiple electrode aggregometry: a new device to measure platelet aggregation in whole blood. *Thromb. Haemost*. 2006;96:781–8.

[12] Van Werkum, J. W., Kleibeuker, M., Postma, S., Bouman, H. J., Elsenberg, E. H., Ten Berg, J. M., et al. A comparison between the Plateletworks-assay and light transmittance aggregometry for monitoring the inhibitory effects of clopidogrel. *Int. J. Cardiol.* 2008;140:123–6.

[13] Malinin, A., Pokov, A., Swaim, L., Kotob, M., Serebruany, V. Validation of a VerifyNow-P2Y12 cartridge for monitoring platelet inhibition with clopidogrel. *Methods Find Exp. Clin. Pharmacol.* 2006; 28:315–22.

[14] Aleil, B., Ravanat, C., Cazenave, J. P., Rochoux, G., Heitz, A., Gachet, C. Flow cytometric analysis of intraplatelet VASP phosphorylation for the detection of clopidogrel resistance in patients with ischemic cardiovascular diseases. *J. Thromb. Haemost*. 2005;3:85–92.

[15] Lordkipanidzé, M., Pharand, C., Nguyen, T. A., Schampaert, E., Palisaitis, D. A., Diodati, J. G. Comparison of four tests to assess

inhibition of platelet function by clopidogrel in stable coronary artery disease patients. *Eur. Heart J.* 2008 Dec;29(23):2877-85.

[16] Brar, S. S., ten Berg, J., Marcucci, R., Price, M. J., Valgimigli, M., Kim, H. S., et al. Impact of platelet reactivity on clinical outcomes after percutaneous coronary intervention: a collaborative meta-analysis of individual participant data. *J. Am. Coll. Cardiol.* 2011;58:1945–54.

[17] Matetzky, S., Shenkman, B., Guetta, V., Shechter, M., Beinart, R., Goldenberg, I., Novikov, I., Pres, H., Savion, N., Varon, D., Hod, H. Clopidogrel resistance is associated with increased risk of recurrent atherothrombotic events in patients with acute myocardial infarction. *Circulation.* 2004 Jun. 29;109(25):3171-5.

[18] Price, M. J., Berger, P. B., Teirstein, P. S., Tanguay, J. F., Angiolillo, D. J., Spriggs, D., Puri, S., Robbins, M., Garratt, K. N., Bertrand, O. F., Stillabower, M. E., Aragon, J. R., Kandzari, D. E., Stinis, C. T., Lee, M. S., Manoukian, S. V., Cannon, C. P., Schork, N. J., Topol, E. J.; GRAVITAS Investigators. Standard- vs high-dose clopidogrel based on platelet function testing after percutaneous coronary intervention: the GRAVITAS randomized trial. *JAMA.* 2011;305(11):1097-1105.

[19] Price, M. J., Angiolillo, D. J., Teirstein, P. S., Lillie, E., Manoukian, S. V., Berger, P. B., et al. Platelet reactivity and cardiovascular outcomes after percutaneous coronary intervention: a time-dependent analysis of the gauging responsiveness with a verifynow P2Y12 assay: impact on thrombosis and safety (GRAVITAS) trial. *Circulation.* 2011;124:1132–7.

[20] Stone, G. W., Witzenbichler, B., Weisz, G., Rinaldi, M. J., Neumann, F. J., Metzger, D. C., Henry, T. D., Cox, D. A., Duffy, P. L., Mazzaferri, E., Gurbel, P. A., Xu, K., Parise, H., Kirtane, A. J., Brodie, B. R., Mehran, R., Stuckey, T. D.; ADAPT-DES Investigators. Platelet reactivity and clinical outcomes after coronary artery implantation of drug-eluting stents (ADAPT-DES): a prospective multicentre registry study. *Lancet.* 2013 Aug. 17;382(9892):614-23. doi: 10.1016/S0140-6736(13)61170-8.

[21] Bonello, L., Camoin-Jau, L., Arques, S., Boyer, C., Panagides, D., Wittenberg, O., Simeoni, M. C., Barragan, P., Dignat-George, F., Paganelli, F. Adjusted clopidogrel loading doses according to vasodilator-stimulated phosphoprotein phosphorylation index decrease rate of major adverse cardiovascular events in patients with clopidogrel resistance: a multicenter randomized prospective study. *J. Am. Coll. Cardiol.* 2008 Apr. 8;51(14):1404-11.

[22] Collet, J. P., Cuisset, T., Rangé, G., Cayla, G., Elhadad, S., Pouillot, C., Henry, P., Motreff, P., Carrié, D., Boueri, Z., Belle, L., Van Belle, E., Rousseau, H., Aubry, P., Monségu, J., Sabouret, P., O'Connor, S. A., Abtan, J., Kerneis, M., Saint-Etienne, C., Barthélémy, O., Beygui, F., Silvain, J., Vicaut, E., Montalescot, G.; ARCTIC Investigators. Bedside monitoring to adjust antiplatelet therapy for coronary stenting. *N. Engl. J. Med.* 2012 Nov. 29;367(22):2100-9.

[23] Valgimigli, M., Campo, G., de Cesare, N., Meliga, E., Vranckx, P., Furgieri, A., et al. Intensifying platelet inhibition with tirofiban in poor responders to aspirin, clopidogrel, or both agents undergoing elective coronary intervention: results from the double-blind, prospective, randomized tailoring treatment with tirofiban in patients showing resistance to aspirin and/or resistance to clopidogrel study. *Circulation.* 2009;119:3215–22.

[24] Trenk, D., Stone, G. W., Gawaz, M., Kastrati, A., Angiolillo, D. J., Muller, U., et al. A randomized trial of prasugrel versus clopidogrel in patients with high platelet reactivity on clopidogrel after elective percutaneous coronary intervention with implantation of drug eluting stents: results of the TRIGGER-PCI (Testing Platelet Reactivity In Patients Undergoing Elective Stent Placement on Clopidogrel to Guide Alternative Therapy With Prasugrel) Study. *J. Am. Coll. Cardiol.* 2012; 59:2159–64.

[25] Levine, G. N., Bates, E. R., Blankenship, J. C., Bailey, S. R., Bittl, J. A., Cercek, B., Chambers, C. E., Ellis, S. G., Guyton, R. A., Hollenberg, S. M., Khot, U. N., Lange, R. A., Mauri, L., Mehran, R., Moussa, I. D., Mukherjee, D., Nallamothu, B. K., Ting, H. H. 2011 ACCF/AHA/SCAI Guideline for Percutaneous Coronary Intervention: executive summary: a report of the American College of Cardiology Foundation/American Heart Association Task Force on Practice Guidelines and the Society for Cardiovascular Angiography and Interventions. *Circulation.* 2011 Dec. 6;124(23):2574-609.

[26] Jneid, H., Anderson, J. L., Wright, R. S., Adams, C. D., Bridges, C. R., Casey, D. E., Jr., et al. 2012 ACCF/AHA focused update of the guideline for the management of patients with unstable angina/non-ST-elevation myocardial infarction (updating the 2007 guideline and replacing the 2011 focused update): a report of the american college of cardiology foundation/american heart association task force on practice guidelines. *Circulation.* 2012;126:875–910.

INDEX

B

C

I

N

O

P

Q

R

S

T

U

V

W

Y